Triage Systems: Essential Knowledge for Emergency Nurses and Physicians

Arian Zaboli · Gianni Turcato

Triage Systems: Essential Knowledge for Emergency Nurses and Physicians

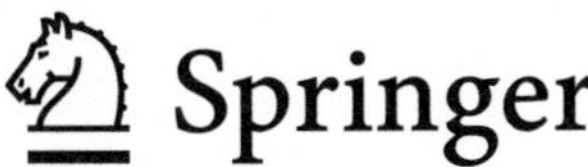

Arian Zaboli
Health Professions Management
South Tyrolean Health Authority
(SABES-ASDAA)
Bolzano, Italy

Gianni Turcato
Internal Medicine
Hospital Alto Vicentino
Santorso VI, Italy

ISBN 978-3-032-20824-8   ISBN 978-3-032-20825-5   (eBook)
https://doi.org/10.1007/978-3-032-20825-5

This Springer imprint is published by the registered company Springer Nature Switzerland AG
The registered company address is: Gewerbestrasse 11, 6330 Cham, Switzerland

If disposing of this product, please recycle the paper.

Preface

Emergency Medicine is a young, dynamic discipline in constant transformation. Precisely for this reason, it is an exceptionally fertile field: every stage of growth requires exploration, innovation, and, above all, critical engagement with evidence. Today, however, this evolutionary momentum confronts a structural crisis in healthcare systems whose most visible point of impact is emergency care. By its very nature, the Emergency Department cannot close, cannot defer access, and cannot postpone demand: it remains the safety net of the system when other levels of care slow down, fragment, or retreat.

Population ageing, increasing frailty and multimorbidity, reduced professional and infrastructural resources in community care, and rising social complexity place sustained pressure on emergency services. This is further compounded by vulnerability: patients without family networks, without social support, and without continuous care pathways. Many arrive not only with clinical needs but also with social and assistance needs that the hospital is not designed to absorb sustainably. In this setting, demand rises, waiting times lengthen, clinical risk increases, and the entire system becomes more exposed to operational failure.

In this context, a simple question becomes unavoidable: why focus on triage? Because triage is not merely an organizational step; it is the mechanism that allows the system to remain functional when resources are not proportional to demand. It is the process that translates complexity into clinical priorities, distinguishing what cannot safely wait from what can be managed with appropriate timing. In practical terms, triage represents the first clinical decision of the Emergency Department: a decision taken under uncertainty, within minutes, with limited information, yet with potentially decisive consequences for the patient's pathway and outcomes.

Effective triage does not simply decide who is seen first. It shapes the entire care trajectory, supports proportional decision-making, mitigates the harm of dangerous delays, contributes to flow management, and, when embedded in a coherent reassessment process, strengthens overall safety. Under conditions of relative scarcity, triage also functions as a concrete form of distributive justice: a transparent, clinically grounded way of assigning priority, ensuring that access is not determined by chance or by "first come, first served."

Despite this, deeply rooted misconceptions persist. Triage is often viewed as a purely executive task confined to the triage nurse, or as an activity that clinical experience alone can replace without structured methodology. These interpretations underestimate the cognitive complexity of triage and diminish its strategic importance. Triage demands clinical competence, communication skills, conflict management, probabilistic thinking, and proficiency with standardized systems. It is not a minor preliminary step, but a high-stakes decision point.

This book was written to help correct these distortions. On the one hand, it aims to place triage back at the center of scientific discussion by clearly defining its principles, historical evolution, operational logic, and evidence base. On the other hand, it seeks to return triage to the entire emergency care system: triage should not be the exclusive domain of the individual professional who performs it, but a shared language for physicians, nurses, and students. The quality of downstream decisions inevitably depends on the quality of the decisions made upstream.

To build a solid foundation, we start from the major internationally validated five-level triage systems, Manchester Triage System (MTS), Emergency Severity Index (ESI), Australasian Triage Scale (ATS), Canadian Triage and Acuity Scale (CTAS), and South African Triage Scale (SATS). These models are not simply successful implementations; they are structured attempts to formalize a complex process, make it reproducible, measurable, and continuously improvable. A wide range of local and national systems also exists, reflecting legitimate efforts to adapt triage to specific contexts. However, at a time when emergency care requires comparability, coherence, and shared progress, engaging critically with validated international systems offers a decisive advantage: it avoids repeatedly starting from zero and supports cumulative scientific development.

An additional objective of this book is to offer international readers a comparative perspective, placing local practice in dialogue with the broader global triage landscape, and to contribute, as far as possible, to a common language for urgency and prioritization across different healthcare systems. Understanding similarities and differences between frameworks is essential for safe implementation, meaningful benchmarking, and informed interpretation of the international literature.

This text does not claim to close the discussion on triage; rather, it aims to open it, make it accessible, and make it useful. By addressing foundations (triage as risk stratification), comparing models, analyzing performance, and identifying what can realistically be improved in the short and long term, the goal is to provide those entering emergency care with a clear and rigorous base. Only through a shared culture, scientific, critical, and operational can triage assume the role it deserves and support Emergency Departments in evolving toward systems that are safer, more effective, and more sustainable.

Bolzano, Italy   Arian Zaboli
Santorso VI, Italy   Gianni Turcato

Contents

Part II   The Current Triage Systems

Part III   The Possible Future of Triage Systems

Part I

The Past of Triage Systems

The Purpose of In-Hospital Triage Systems in the Emergency Department

1

The concept of triage has its roots in the dramatic context of warfare, where the need to manage large numbers of wounded individuals with drastically limited medical resources compelled the development of systematic methodologies for the rapid and accurate selection of patients according to the severity of their conditions and their probabilities of survival [1, 2]. The term derives from the French verb "trier," meaning "to select" or "to separate," and is traditionally attributed to the pioneering work of the French military surgeon Dominique Jean Larrey during the Napoleonic campaigns at the end of the eighteenth century [1, 2].

Larrey, chief surgeon of Napoleon's Grande Armée, revolutionized military medicine by introducing systematic principles for the prioritization of the wounded. His methodological innovation lay in establishing priority criteria not on the basis of military or social rank, as was customary at the time, but solely according to the severity of injuries and the likelihood of immediate benefit from medical treatment [1–3]. This approach, seemingly simple yet revolutionary for its era, stipulated that those with the highest probability of survival if treated promptly should be managed first, followed by those with less severe injuries who could safely wait, while cases deemed irrecoverable were provided only with palliative care [2, 3].

The underlying logic of this system, rapidly deciding who requires immediate treatment, who can safely wait, and who needs only comfort care, progressively consolidated through successive military experiences of the nineteenth and twentieth centuries [4]. During the American Civil War (1861–1865), the Franco-Prussian War (1870–1871), and subsequently throughout the two World Wars, the principles of military triage were refined and systematized, giving rise to modern methodologies for mass-casualty management and inspiring the development of contemporary emergency response organization in situations with a high number of victims [2, 5, 6].

The experience accumulated in armed conflicts highlighted several fundamental principles that remain valid today: the need for rapid decisions based on objective criteria; the importance of specific training for healthcare personnel; the centrality

© The Author(s), under exclusive license to Springer Nature
Switzerland AG 2026
A. Zaboli, G. Turcato, *Triage Systems: Essential Knowledge for Emergency Nurses and Physicians*, https://doi.org/10.1007/978-3-032-20825-5_1

of documentation for monitoring and continuous improvement; and, above all, the ethical principle of "the greatest good for the greatest number" in contexts of resource scarcity [4, 7].

For many decades after its initial codification, triage remained predominantly associated with "in-the-field" management of military and civilian mass emergencies [2, 3]. However, beginning in the mid-twentieth century, and with particular intensity between the 1950s and 1960s, the concept began to find systematic application within civilian hospitals, in response to demographic, epidemiological, and organizational changes that were radically transforming the landscape of emergency medicine [8–10].

The post-war period was characterized by profound social and economic changes that significantly influenced the demand for emergency medical care. Accelerated urbanization, increased individual mobility, the development of the automotive industry with the consequent rise in road traffic accidents, and changes in lifestyles all contributed to an exponential increase in attendances at hospitals Emergency Departments [9, 11].

The United States, Canada, the United Kingdom, and Western Europe recorded increases in emergency department attendances far exceeding the response capacity of existing healthcare facilities [12–14]. In the United States, for example, the number of visits to emergency departments rose by 300% between 1940 and 1960, while hospital capacity expanded by only 50% [15, 16]. This imbalance created conditions of chronic overcrowding that compromised the quality and safety of care, particularly for the most critical patients [17, 18].

The introduction of in-hospital triage constituted a systematic response to this growing pressure, establishing structured methodologies for the prioritization of interventions and ensuring that critical cases received care within time frames commensurate with clinical risk [19–21]. In those pioneering years, hospital triage often consisted of a rapid clinical assessment at the Emergency Department entrance, aimed primarily at determining the order of medical evaluation in the context of limited resources [19–21].

Early hospital triage systems were characterized by operational simplicity and a predominantly intuitive approach, grounded in the clinical experience of healthcare personnel [19–21]. Nevertheless, even at this embryonic stage, several methodological principles emerged that would become fundamental to the development of modern systems: the need for standardized criteria, the importance of specific staff training, and the centrality of documentation for performance monitoring [22].

1.1 Fundamental Characteristics of Modern In-Hospital Triage

The evolution of in-hospital triage has led to the definition of a structured methodology with specific characteristics that distinguish it from other forms of clinical assessment [22]. The implementation of modern triage at the entrance to emergency departments is founded on several core principles that ensure operational effectiveness and clinical safety [20–22].

Rapidity is an indispensable requirement of the triage process [23]. The assessment must be completed in a very short time, typically within 5 min per patient, to prevent the process itself from becoming a bottleneck in patient flow [24]. This timeliness is essential to ensure that critically ill patients receive immediate attention and that the system can effectively manage surges in demand [24].

However, the speed of triage must not compromise the accuracy of the assessment [24]. Modern systems have developed structured methodologies that make it possible to obtain clinically relevant information in a very short time through the use of decision algorithms, standardized assessment scales, and specific protocols [25].

Triage is characterized by an essentialist approach based on a brief, targeted history, direct clinical observation, and measurement of fundamental vital signs, without recourse to instrumental diagnostics [21, 26]. This essentiality is necessary to maintain the speed of the process, but it requires high-level clinical competence on the part of the practitioner to maximize diagnostic effectiveness with limited means [21, 26].

History-taking in triage focuses on key elements: the primary reason for attendance, duration and mode of symptom onset, pain intensity, the presence of known risk factors, and any similar previous episodes [22, 27, 28]. Clinical observation concentrates on immediately assessable aspects: level of consciousness, skin color, respiratory pattern, posture, ability to ambulate, signs of distress, and finally vital signs.

The stratification of patients into urgency levels represents the core of the triage process [22, 27, 28]. Patients are divided into categories that define target times for medical evaluation, ensuring priority access for the most severe and allowing safe waiting for the less critical. This stratification must be based on objective and reproducible clinical criteria to guarantee fairness and consistency in decision-making [22, 27, 28].

Target times do not constitute rigid limits but operational benchmarks that enable performance monitoring of the system and the identification of problematic situations.

1.2   Primary Function of In-Hospital Triage

The primary function of triage in the hospital setting is to protect the patient from the potentially devastating effects of delays in accessing appropriate care [22, 28]. In an emergency department, where true emergencies coexist with non-urgent healthcare needs, the ability to correctly identify and prioritize critical patients constitutes a clinical, ethical, and organizational imperative of fundamental importance [29].

Treating the most severely ill patients first is not only an operational necessity but also a fundamental ethical imperative that reflects the basic principles of medicine: primum non nocere and beneficence. Triage enables scarce resources to be allocated efficiently and fairly, significantly reducing the risk of preventable adverse events and optimizing overall clinical outcomes [30].

The ethical dimension of triage has been the subject of extensive philosophical and bioethical analysis [3, 31]. The system safeguards fundamental values such as life, health, the efficient use of public resources, and equity in access to care [3, 31]. It requires healthcare professionals to make rapid, informed decisions under conditions of uncertainty, recognizing that inaction or delayed decision-making may represent the worst option in terms of clinical outcomes [4].

Triage embodies the principles of distributive justice as applied to emergency medicine. In situations of relative resource scarcity, the system ensures that the allocation of care follows objective clinical criteria rather than irrelevant factors such as social status, economic means, or order of arrival. This function is particularly important in public healthcare systems, where equitable access represents a core value.

The transparency of triage criteria is essential to maintain public trust in the healthcare system and to ensure that decisions can be understood and accepted by patients and their families [3, 4, 31].

1.3   Dynamics of Flows in the Emergency Department

The functioning of an emergency department can be conceptualized as a dynamic system characterized by continuous, interdependent flows that determine overall efficiency and the quality of care delivered [32]. This systemic perspective is essential to understand the strategic role of triage in optimizing department performance.

The conceptual model most commonly used to describe the operational dynamics of an emergency department identifies three main flows [33, 34]:

Input: represents the entry of patients into the system. It is characterized by high temporal variability, unpredictability, and heterogeneity of clinical conditions. Input is influenced by external factors such as seasonality, weather events, epidemics, mass-casualty incidents, and local socio-economic dynamics.

Throughput: encompasses all clinical-care processes that take place within the emergency department, from the initial assessment to the decision to discharge or admit. It includes triage, medical evaluation, diagnostic investigations, treatments, specialist consultations, and clinical observation.

Output: represents patients leaving the system through discharge home, hospital admission, transfer to other facilities, or death. The efficiency of output is often influenced by factors external to the emergency department, such as bed availability, the efficiency of inpatient wards, and the capacity of the community network.

The balance among these three flows is determined by the resources available and the system's ability to provide continuous care. In clinical practice, throughput is often "compressed" by high input or by difficulties in output (for example, bed shortages for admission), generating congestion phenomena that may compromise the quality and safety of care [33, 34].

Even an intrinsically efficient emergency department can rapidly reach saturation if output mechanisms become blocked or slow significantly [35, 36]. This dynamic, known as "boarding" or "bed blocking," represents one of the main operational challenges for modern emergency departments and requires systemic strategies to be addressed effectively [35, 36].

Within this systemic context, triage, strategically positioned at the beginning of the care pathway, acts as a multifunctional clinical-organizational filter. It mitigates the impact of unpredictable arrivals, directs clinical attention promptly toward patients at highest risk, and facilitates the optimization of internal flows through early streaming toward appropriate care pathways (Fig. 1.1).

Triage cannot control input, which remains largely unpredictable, but it can significantly influence throughput efficiency through accurate prioritization and intelligent streaming [33–35]. This function becomes particularly critical during demand peaks, when system capacity is under maximal stress [33–35].

Among the three flows that characterize the functioning of an emergency department, input is the most difficult to govern due to two intrinsic features that distinguish it from other healthcare services: open access and unpredictability [34, 37].

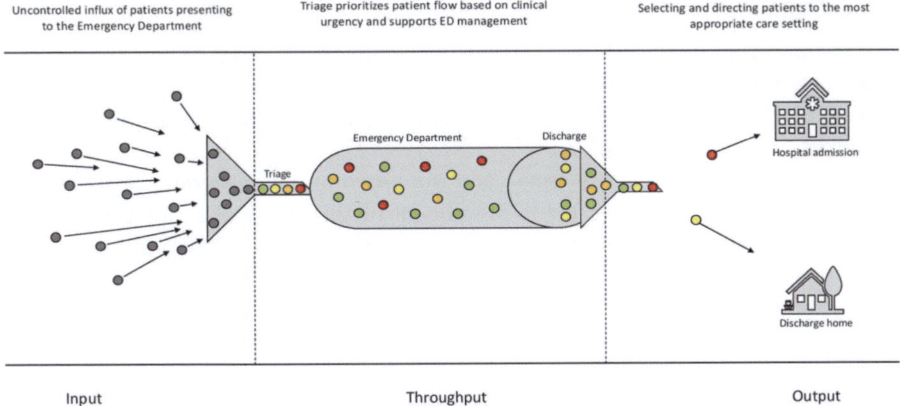

Fig. 1.1 Input–Throughput–Output model of Emergency Department flow and the role of triage. The input phase reflects an uncontrolled influx of patients presenting to the ED (grey dots). At triage, patients are rapidly assessed and prioritized according to clinical urgency (colored dots), enabling safer allocation of time and resources and supporting ED flow management. During the throughput phase, patients progress through evaluation and treatment within the ED while awaiting a final disposition decision. The output phase represents patient selection and routing to the most appropriate care setting, typically hospital admission or discharge home. Color code: red = highest clinical emergency/high risk; orange = high urgency; yellow = intermediate urgency; green = lower urgency/low immediate risk. Dashed vertical lines separate the three phases

The principle of open access establishes that anyone may present to an emergency department at any time, without an appointment, referral, or prior authorization. While fundamental to guaranteeing universal access to emergency care, this principle generates significant operational challenges for planning and resource allocation.

Open access entails that the emergency department must be constantly prepared to manage any type of emergency, from the most common to the rarest and most complex, without the possibility of prior scheduling. This feature requires organizational flexibility, resource redundancy, and the capacity for rapid adaptation to fluctuations in demand.

The unpredictability of input represents an even more complex challenge. Despite decades of epidemiological research and the development of sophisticated statistical models, no tools exist that can accurately predict when and how many patients will arrive at an emergency department, nor what the severity and complexity mix of their conditions will be [38, 39].

This unpredictability manifests across different temporal scales: hourly variations, daily variations, seasonal variations, and exceptional variations linked to unforeseen events (mass-casualty incidents, public health emergencies, and extreme weather events) [40].

Triage allows at least part of this variability to be absorbed through mechanisms of dynamic compensation [41]. It places patients with signs of clinical instability in "pole position," ensuring them priority access regardless of the overall volume of arrivals [41]. At the same time, it enables safe waiting for less critical patients, with the possibility of dynamically reassessing priority if clinical conditions change during the wait.

This buffering function is particularly important during demand peaks, when the system operates near saturation. Triage ensures that, even under conditions of maximal operational stress, the most critical patients maintain priority access to available resources [22, 28].

The operational success of triage and the growing understanding of its importance for patient safety have led to significant methodological evolution. Starting from the 1990s, triage has progressively consolidated into structured, evidence-based systems characterized by rigorous standardization and scientific validation [42].

1.4   Transition to Evidence-Based Triage

The transition from empirical to structured systems was driven by the need to overcome the limitations of the early approaches to hospital triage: high inter-operator variability, lack of objective criteria, difficulties in performance monitoring, and limited capacity for audit and continuous improvement [25, 43].

Modern structured systems are characterized by explicit, standardized assessment criteria; uniform priority scales with defined target times; specific training protocols for practitioners; audit and quality assurance mechanisms; and integration with information systems for performance monitoring [43, 44].

All modern, validated triage systems adopt a five-level priority structure, which represents the best compromise between clinical granularity and operational practicability [43–45]. This standardization facilitates comparability across different institutions, staff training, and the development of scientific research in the field of triage. Each level is associated with specific target times for medical evaluation and with standardized clinical criteria for assignment [44].

Despite the significant benefits documented in the scientific literature, the implementation and maintenance of effective triage systems present certain critical issues that require constant attention and targeted mitigation strategies.

1.5   Streaming and Triage

Within the management of flows in emergency departments, it is essential to draw a clear distinction between two processes which, although often used interchangeably in everyday practice, have substantially different characteristics, objectives, and methodologies: triage and streaming. Beyond its theoretical relevance, this distinction has particular practical importance in designing effective organizational systems and optimizing care pathways.

Triage, as previously discussed, is a systematic process of clinical assessment aimed at stratifying patients according to clinical priority and urgency of treatment [43–45]. Its primary objective is to rapidly identify patients who require immediate medical intervention, distinguishing them from those who can safely wait without risk of clinical deterioration [43, 45]. Triage is therefore essentially a temporal prioritization process based on standardized clinical criteria [43, 45].

Streaming, by contrast, is an organizational routing process that directs patients toward the most appropriate care pathway on the basis of their clinical characteristics, the type of problem presented, and the resources available within the Department [46, 47]. The objective of streaming is not to establish temporal priority, but to identify the optimal care setting for each patient, thereby optimizing resource utilization and reducing overall throughput times [46, 48].

Streaming represents a natural complement to traditional triage alone. It does not merely assign a temporal priority to patients but aims to direct each patient early toward the care pathway most suited to their specific clinical complexity and care needs (Fig. 1.2).

Streaming is founded on the principle that patients with similar clinical characteristics and care needs can be managed more effectively through dedicated, optimized pathways [46, 48]. This approach prevents overloading specialist resources with low-intensity needs while simultaneously freeing capacity for the management of true emergencies. It is important to note that, unlike triage, streaming depends significantly on the hospital context and on the structure and local healthcare network, whereas triage is based on evidence-based indications and standardized systems.

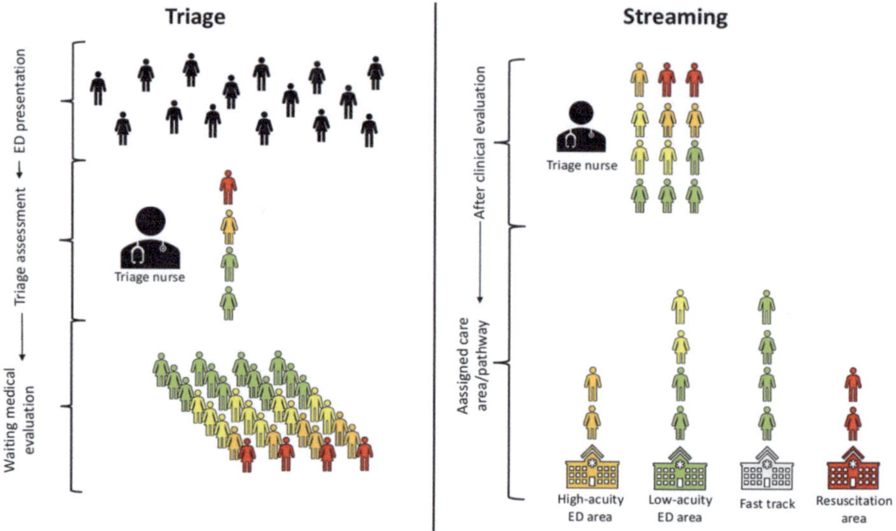

Fig. 1.2 Conceptual distinction between triage and streaming in the emergency department. In triage (left panel), patients presenting to the ED undergo a rapid triage assessment and are prioritized in time according to clinical urgency/acuity: higher-acuity patients are placed earlier in the queue for medical evaluation, while lower-acuity patients may safely wait, with reassessment as needed. In streaming (right panel), after the same initial assessment, patients are assigned to the most appropriate ED care area or pathway based on urgency and expected care needs/resources (e.g., resuscitation area, high-acuity area, low-acuity area, or fast-track/minor injury pathway). Thus, triage primarily answers "who should be seen first?", whereas streaming answers "where should the patient be managed?"; in practice, both processes can be integrated to improve safety and patient flow. Color code: red = highest clinical emergency/high risk; orange = high urgency; yellow = intermediate urgency; green = lower urgency/low immediate risk

References

1. Turner MD, Shah MH. Dominique-Jean Larrey (1766-1842): the founder of the modern triage system. Cureus. 2024;16(6):e62375. https://doi.org/10.7759/cureus.62375.
2. Iserson KV, Moskop JC. Triage in medicine, part I: concept, history, and types. Ann Emerg Med. 2007;49(3):275–81. https://doi.org/10.1016/j.annemergmed.2006.05.019. Epub 2006 Jul 10
3. Moskop JC, Iserson KV. Triage in medicine, part II: underlying values and principles. Ann Emerg Med. 2007;49(3):282–7. https://doi.org/10.1016/j.annemergmed.2006.07.012. Epub 2006 Aug 14
4. Ferrara A. The ethical triage dilemma: who should receive medical care first; is this the right question? Ratio Juris. 2023;36(2):178–90. https://doi.org/10.1111/raju.12376.
5. Nakao H, Ukai I, Kotani J. A review of the history of the origin of triage from a disaster medicine perspective. Acute Med Surg. 2017;4(4):379–84. https://doi.org/10.1002/ams2.293.
6. Pollock RA. Triage and management of the injured in world war I: the diuturnity of antoine de page and a belgian colleague. Craniomaxillofac Trauma Reconstr. 2008;1(1):63–70. https://doi.org/10.1055/s-0028-1098965.
7. Christ M, Grossmann F, Winter D, Bingisser R, Platz E. Modern triage in the emergency department. Dtsch Arztebl Int. 2010;107(50):892–8. https://doi.org/10.3238/arztebl.2010.0892. Epub 2010 Dec 17

8. Özdemir S. A brief overview of the application of triage systems in the emergency department during pandemic period. Maltepe Med J. 2022;14(1):28–9. https://doi.org/10.35514/mtd.2022.65.

9. Merritt AK. The rise of emergency medicine in the sixties: paving a new entrance to the house of medicine. J Hist Med Allied Sci. 2014;69(2):251–93. https://doi.org/10.1093/jhmas/jrs054. Epub 2012 Sep 10

10. American College of Emergency Physicians, Subcommittee on National Triage Scale, Emergency Medicine Practice Committee. A uniform triage scale in emergency medicine [information paper]. Dallas (TX): American College of Emergency Physicians; 1999.

11. National Academy of Sciences; National Research Council, Committee on Trauma and Committee on Shock. Accidental death and disability: the neglected disease of modern society. Washington (DC): National Academy of Sciences; 1966.

12. Schull MJ, Slaughter PM, Redelmeier DA. Urban emergency department overcrowding: defining the problem and eliminating misconceptions. CJEM. 2002;4(2):76–83. https://doi.org/10.1017/s1481803500006163.

13. Higginson I, Boyle A. What should we do about crowding in emergency departments? Br J Hosp Med (Lond). 2018;79(9):500–3. https://doi.org/10.12968/hmed.2018.79.9.500.

14. Morley C, Unwin M, Peterson GM, Stankovich J, Kinsman L. Emergency department crowding: a systematic review of causes, consequences and solutions. PLoS One. 2018;13(8):e0203316. https://doi.org/10.1371/journal.pone.0203316.

15. Zink BJ. Social justice, egalitarianism, and the history of emergency medicine. Virtual Mentor. 2010;12(6):492–4.

16. American Hospital Association. Emergency services: the hospital emergency department in an emergency care system. Chicago (IL): American Hospital Association; 1972.

17. Institute of Medicine. Hospital-based emergency care: at the breaking point. Washington (DC): National Academies Press; 2007.

18. Trzeciak S, Rivers EP. Emergency department overcrowding in the United States: an emerging threat to patient safety and public health. Emerg Med J. 2003;20(5):402–5.

19. Department of Health and Ageing. Emergency triage education kit: resource book. Canberra: Commonwealth of Australia; 2009.

20. Jelinek GA. Triage: coming of age. Emerg Med Australas. 2008;20(3):196–8. https://doi.org/10.1111/j.1742-6723.2008.01091.x.

21. Yancey CC, O'Rourke MC. Emergency Department Triage. 2023. In: StatPearls [Internet]. Treasure Island (FL): StatPearls Publishing; 2025.

22. FitzGerald G, Jelinek GA, Scott D, Gerdtz MF. Emergency department triage revisited. Emerg Med J. 2010;27(2):86–92. https://doi.org/10.1136/emj.2009.077081.

23. Hitchcock M, Gillespie B, Crilly J, Chaboyer W. Triage: an investigation of the process and potential vulnerabilities. J Adv Nurs. 2014;70(7):1532–41. https://doi.org/10.1111/jan.12304. Epub 2013 Dec 23

24. Zaboli A, Brigo F, Brigiari G, Massar M, Pfeifer N, Turcato G. Beyond nurse efficiency: a multilevel analysis of nurse, contextual, and patient-related factors in triage duration. J Emerg Nurs. 2025;51(5):816–825.e2. https://doi.org/10.1016/j.jen.2025.04.008. Epub 2025 May 19

25. Tam HL, Chung SF, Lou CK. A review of triage accuracy and future direction. BMC Emerg Med. 2018;18(1):58. https://doi.org/10.1186/s12873-018-0215-0.

26. Sapra A, Malik A, Bhandari P. Vital sign assessment. In: StatPearls [Internet]. Treasure Island (FL): StatPearls Publishing; 2025. Updated 2023 Jul 24.

27. Gilboy N, Tanabe T, Travers D, Rosenau AM, Eitel DR. Emergency severity index (ESI), version 4: implementation handbook. Rockville (MD): Agency for Healthcare Research and Quality; 2005. AHRQ Publication No. 05-0046-2

28. Australasian College for Emergency Medicine. Guidelines on the implementation of the Australasian Triage Scale in Emergency Departments. Melbourne: ACEM; 2023. (G24, Version 6). acem.org.au

29. Zaboli A, Turcato G, Brigiari G, Massar M, Ziller M, Sibilio S, Brigo F. Emergency departments in contemporary healthcare: are they still for emergencies? An analysis of over 1 million attendances. Healthcare (Basel). 2024;12(23):2426. https://doi.org/10.3390/healthcare12232426.
30. Challen K. How good is triage, and what is it good for? Emerg Med J. 2017;34(11):702. https://doi.org/10.1136/emermed-2017-206973. Epub 2017 Oct 4
31. Aacharya RP, Gastmans C, Denier Y. Emergency department triage: an ethical analysis. BMC Emerg Med. 2011;11:16. https://doi.org/10.1186/1471-227X-11-16.
32. Samadbeik M, Staib A, Boyle J, Khanna S, Bosley E, Bodnar D, Lind J, Austin JA, Tanner S, Meshkat Y, de Courten B, Sullivan C. Patient flow in emergency departments: a comprehensive umbrella review of solutions and challenges across the health system. BMC Health Serv Res. 2024;24(1):274. https://doi.org/10.1186/s12913-024-10725-6.
33. Savioli G, Ceresa IF, Gri N, Bavestrello Piccini G, Longhitano Y, Zanza C, Piccioni A, Esposito C, Ricevuti G, Bressan MA. Emergency department overcrowding: understanding the factors to find corresponding solutions. J Pers Med. 2022;12(2):279. https://doi.org/10.3390/jpm12020279.
34. Asplin BR, Magid DJ, Rhodes KV, Solberg LI, Lurie N, Camargo CA Jr. A conceptual model of emergency department crowding. Ann Emerg Med. 2003;42(2):173–80. https://doi.org/10.1067/mem.2003.302.
35. Kelen GD, Wolfe R, D'Onofrio G, et al. Emergency department crowding: the canary in the health care system. NEJM Catal Innov Care Deliv. 2021; https://doi.org/10.1056/CAT.21.0217.
36. Sartini M, Carbone A, Demartini A, Giribone L, Oliva M, Spagnolo AM, Cremonesi P, Canale F, Cristina ML. Overcrowding in emergency department: causes, consequences, and solutions-a narrative review. Healthcare (Basel). 2022;10(9):1625. https://doi.org/10.3390/healthcare10091625.
37. Boyle AA, Beniuk K. Overcrowding: emergency departments are the canary in the coal mine and overcrowding is the poisonous gas. Eur J Emerg Med. 2010;17(6):354. https://doi.org/10.1097/MEJ.0b013e32833821e5.
38. Weiss SJ, Derlet R, Arndahl J, Ernst AA, Richards J, Fernández-Frackelton M, Schwab R, Stair TO, Vicellio P, Levy D, Brautigan M, Johnson A, Nick TG. Estimating the degree of emergency department overcrowding in academic medical centers: results of the National ED Overcrowding Study (NEDOCS). Acad Emerg Med. 2004;11(1):38–50. https://doi.org/10.1197/j.aem.2003.07.017. Erratum in: Acad Emerg Med. 2004;11(4):408. Fernández-Frankelton M [corrected to Fernández-Frackelton M].
39. Hwang U, McCarthy ML, Aronsky D, Asplin B, Crane PW, Craven CK, Epstein SK, Fee C, Handel DA, Pines JM, Rathlev NK, Schafermeyer RW, Zwemer FL Jr, Bernstein SL. Measures of crowding in the emergency department: a systematic review. Acad Emerg Med. 2011;18(5):527–38. https://doi.org/10.1111/j.1553-2712.2011.01054.x.
40. Zaboli A, Brigo F, Brigiari G, Turcato G. Exploring the variability in triage nursing workload: insights from a multicentre observational study. J Adv Nurs. 2025;81(8):4690–7. https://doi.org/10.1111/jan.16627. Epub 2024 Nov 12
41. Agency for Healthcare Research and Quality. Emergency severity index (ESI): a triage tool for emergency department care. Version 4. Implementation handbook. Rockville (MD): AHRQ; 2012.
42. Robertson-Steel I. Evolution of triage systems. Emerg Med J. 2006;23(2):154–5. https://doi.org/10.1136/emj.2005.030270.
43. Zachariasse JM, van der Hagen V, Seiger N, Mackway-Jones K, van Veen M, Moll HA. Performance of triage systems in emergency care: a systematic review and meta-analysis. BMJ Open. 2019;9(5):e026471. https://doi.org/10.1136/bmjopen-2018-026471.
44. Kuriyama A, Urushidani S, Nakayama T. Five-level emergency triage systems: variation in assessment of validity. Emerg Med J. 2017;34(11):703–10. https://doi.org/10.1136/emermed-2016-206295. Epub 2017 Jul 27

45. Hinson JS, Martinez DA, Cabral S, George K, Whalen M, Hansoti B, Levin S. Triage performance in emergency medicine: a systematic review. Ann Emerg Med. 2019;74(1):140–52. https://doi.org/10.1016/j.annemergmed.2018.09.022. Epub 2018 Nov 22
46. Kelly AM, Bryant M, Cox L, Jolley D. Improving emergency department efficiency by patient streaming to outcomes-based teams. Aust Health Rev. 2007;31(1):16–21. https://doi.org/10.1071/ah070016.
47. Saghafian S, Hopp WJ, Van Oyen MP, Desmond JS, Kronick SL. Patient streaming as a mechanism for improving responsiveness in emergency departments. Oper Res. 2012;60(5):1080–97. https://doi.org/10.1287/opre.1120.1096.
48. Anwar MR, Rowe BH, Metge C, Star ND, Aboud Z, Kreindler SA. Realist analysis of streaming interventions in emergency departments. BMJ Leader. 2021;5(3):167–73. https://doi.org/10.1136/leader-2020-000369.

Risk Stratification 2

Risk stratification in contemporary emergency medicine is no longer a refined extension of clinical judgment; it is its backbone, the methodological grammar that allows the clinician to transform bedside observation into a predictive estimate of course and outcomes [1–3]. What makes it so central is not only the inherent uncertainty of emergency care and the need to translate uncertainty into forecasts but also the context in which it is practiced: ever-growing demand for care faced with resources that are often rigid and insufficient. Within this structural tension of abundant need and scarce means arises the clinical and organizational requirement to establish priorities not only by current severity but also by the probability of deterioration and the risk of adverse outcomes if timely action is not taken [4, 5]. Against this backdrop, risk stratification in emergency medicine, and particularly at triage, becomes a methodical response to the problem of distributing clinical attention, time, and resources rationally. What began as an individual act becomes a system process grounded in shared, reproducible criteria aimed at estimating a single patient's risk: risk of serious disease, of rapid deterioration, of high resource utilization, or of death [4, 5]. If we accept that urgency is a function of time and the risk of deterioration, it becomes obvious that a mere "snapshot" of a symptom or condition cannot support robust decisions. To stratify risk is to transform assessment into prediction: a synthetic exercise that orders need, directs diagnostic suspicion, and guides decision-making [6, 7]. In so doing, it bridges the gap between present-moment assessment and eventual outcome, projecting today's observations toward the "after." In triage, this approach turns the first contact into not only a classificatory moment but also a predictive one, capable of identifying those most likely to experience unfavorable outcomes [6, 7]. Literature and organizational practice converge in viewing ED entry as time zero of a progressively intense decision chain, in which anticipating risk is a condition for safety, appropriateness, and continuity. The result is a model that integrates triage and stratification: the former as the operational tool that converts risk estimates into care pathways, the latter as the organizing principle of prediction.

A. Zaboli, G. Turcato, *Triage Systems: Essential Knowledge for Emergency Nurses and Physicians*, https://doi.org/10.1007/978-3-032-20825-5_2

2.1 The Concept and Meaning of Risk Stratification

Risk stratification is a cognitive and operational process by which a graded probability of adverse outcome within a defined time horizon is assigned to a patient, symptom, or clinical condition, and that estimate is used to direct priorities, investigations, and interventions [8]. It is among the most consequential innovations in modern medicine because it transforms clinical observation into predictive evaluation, grouping patients or populations by their risk of critical events and thereby guiding clinical decisions and resource allocation more rationally [8–10]. Brought to the pivotal moment of triage, this perspective implies that the initial assessment is not merely the measurement of signs, vital parameters, or impressions; rather, it is an integration of information that searches for predictive regularities, combines lived clinical experience with risk models, weights variables, and produces, explicitly or implicitly, an estimate of the probability of events such as deterioration, need for critical treatments, admission, readmission, or death [6, 7, 11]. The difference from simple temporal priority is substantial. Priority says who should be seen first; stratification explains why and what the likely consequences are if that does not happen. Priority organizes flow; stratification orients the clinical path. Priority answers a management question; stratification answers a safety question. Once we acknowledge that clinical urgency is not absolute but depends on a patient's biological and functional context, risk stratification becomes the language with which thresholds of attention are defined and monitoring intensity is differentially modulated [12, 13]. Epistemologically, this is akin to the shift from diagnosis as a label to diagnosis as probability: in the ED, decisions are made under time pressure and uncertainty, so each decision is ultimately an informed bet on the likelihood of a clinical state of the world [12, 13]. Risk stratification gives structure to that bet, making it less dependent on momentary heuristics and more anchored to codified experiential rules, validated early signals, and parameters that, combined, increase our ability to foresee evolution [2, 12]. Risk stratification is therefore both a clinical and an organizational operation. Clinical, because it guides the choice to place a patient in a given category and clarifies thresholds for activating time-dependent pathways or for safely adopting abbreviated work-ups. Organizational, because it enables the management of patient flow, the differentiation of pathways, and the allocation of scarce resources to situations with the greatest return in avoided harm and prevented adverse outcomes. Precisely at this crossroads of clinic and organization we see why stratification underpins triage: no order of priorities can stand without a hierarchy of risk, and no hierarchy of risk can be enacted without a device that operationalizes real-time differentiation.

2.2 Why Is It Fundamental at Triage?

Emergency decisions are early, data-poor, time-compressed, and bias-prone. The most costly error is not only diagnostic but prognostic: failing to recognize who will deteriorate as opposed to who, with a similar presentation, can safely wait [14].

Stratification reduces this risk by systematizing what would otherwise be left to intuition: it identifies risk patterns, detects faint signals of physiopathologic derangement, and elevates often-overlooked factors by blending them into a multidimensional picture. In the ED this yields three effects: anticipating deterioration, optimizing resource use, and increasing decision safety [6, 7, 14]. To stratify is to direct interventions first toward those most likely to worsen and to manage lower-risk patients through alternative pathways, reducing overload and inefficiency [15, 16]. It is also a form of clinical justice: priorities are grounded in the true probability of harm, not the appearance of urgency. A risk-oriented assessment helps prevent instability, shortens time-to-care for the most vulnerable, and clarifies who may be discharged with follow-up versus who needs observation or admission. In the window between triage and first physician assessment, stratification acts as an early signaler of time-dependent conditions and guides serial monitoring and checks, making thresholds more transparent and defensible, pathways more coherent, and alignment between clinical intent and action more solid [17, 18]. Finally, it reframes the relationship between symptom and priority: the same clinical sign carries different weight depending on biological substrate and functional reserve; maturity in emergency care lies in anticipating trajectory, not just reacting to the sign.

2.3   Stratification as a Professional Skill in the Emergency Department

Talking about risk stratification is also talking about competencies. Stratification is a composite skill that involves clinical judgment, critical use of predictive tools, the capacity to integrate heterogeneous data under time pressure, contextual sensitivity, and uncertainty management [11, 19]. It is a competency that must belong to everyone working in emergency care, starting with the triage nurse who, before anyone else, must synthesize within minutes a judgment that is faithful to the presentation and sensitive to vulnerability factors [19–21]. Every ED decision, from assigning a triage code to choosing the diagnostic-therapeutic path, from short observation management to the discharge/admit decision, rests on a probabilistic estimate of a future event: risk of deterioration, complication, adverse event, or system overload [21–23]. Risk evaluation is not a one-off act but a continuous process accompanying each phase of care, from initial triage to first clinical assessment to the final disposition [21–23]. It translates clinical complexity into operational priorities, balancing an individual patient's needs with available resources. In this sense, the ability to predict risk is the hallmark of emergency professionalism, the trait that turns reactive intervention into proactive action [21–23]. Whereas other settings focus on diagnosis or treatment, emergency medicine prioritizes uncertainty management. The professional does not only ask "what does the patient have?" but "how likely is the patient to worsen?" this shift, eminently prognostic, permits timely, proportionate decisions. Over the years, this attitude has been formalized into tools and methods: from triage systems to risk scores for specific conditions [21, 24, 25]. These instruments do not replace clinical judgment; they structure it, making it more uniform, shared, and reproducible. Risk thus becomes not an abstract concept but an operational parameter, a common language for methodically handling complexity. In parallel, stratification is also an organizational competency. In a system with finite resources, knowing how to identify and grade risk ensures equity and appropriateness by modulating interventions according to priority. Offering the same level of attention to all is neither possible nor correct: the goal is to guarantee each person the intensity of care their condition demands, as quickly and as safely as possible. Ultimately, risk stratification as a professional skill encapsulates the culture of prediction that permeates emergency medicine: it requires marrying speed with depth, intuition with method, and the individual with the system [21, 24, 25]. It is the competency that protects the patient, sustains service sustainability, and expresses the most authentic cognitive maturity of the contemporary ED.

2.4 Stratification and Triage: Foundational Bond Without Overlap

The relationship between risk stratification and triage is often misunderstood when one imagines the former can replace the latter, or the latter can fully exhaust the former. In reality, triage is the way a system translates a hierarchy of urgency into times and pathways, while stratification is the logic that gives those times and pathways their prognostic meaning [26, 27]. Triage rests on priority; priority rests on risk [26, 27]. If triage were to rank order solely by symptom intensity, it would forfeit much of what determines outcomes; if stratification remained a purely mental exercise not translated into concrete pathways, it would yield no measurable benefit. The meeting point, then, is a triage that is informed by stratification from the first contact and stratification that, from the outset, includes times and modes of reassessment coherent with ED reality. Scientific progress has enabled the move from static triage to triage that incorporates risk awareness as a deep criterion for pathway differentiation [28, 29]. This does not mean overburdening the initial act with complex procedures, but recognizing that certain pieces of information have such prognostic value that they must be gathered immediately and weighed in the decision.

The main protagonist of risk prediction in emergency medicine is the act of triage itself [26, 27]. It is the first clinical act by which the health system meets the acutely ill patient and converts their presentation into an immediate estimate of priority, steering times, pathways, and intensity of care [30]. Triage is therefore not a mere sorting procedure but a true operation of risk stratification. Unfortunately, in common perception, triage is sometimes seen as a purely organizational step. In reality, it is the first and most important clinical forecast along the care path [31]. It must distinguish between those who can safely wait and those who may deteriorate rapidly [31]. The initial evaluation thus becomes the reading of a clinical trajectory, not a simple snapshot. Urgency is not static; it is a function of risk. To stratify is therefore to anticipate what may happen, not only to describe what is already present.

Triage thereby assumes an ethical as well as clinical role: it distributes a scarce good, time, to those who will benefit from it most [20]. The capacity to foresee deterioration is not a methodological accessory; it is the condition that guarantees equity and safety. The evolution of risk stratification has proceeded in parallel with the evolution of triage. The growing complexity of patients and presentations has driven the transition from three- or four-level systems to the widespread adoption of five-level models capable of expressing finer gradations of risk [20, 32, 33]. This increased granularity reflects a conceptual transformation: classification is not just ordering but probabilistic [34]. On it depends not only patient well-being but also departmental efficiency and the sustainability of the entire system.

A decisive function of triage is converting clinical complexity into a shared operational language. Classification transforms myriad symptoms and clinical nuances into a handful of common symbols that allow clinicians, even across systems or countries, to communicate uniformly about severity [20, 27, 28]. Triage thus becomes a systemic translator: from the semantic chaos of reality to a clinical taxonomy that enables rapid decisions [20, 30]. When stratification works, it yields tangible effects. It boosts clinical safety by anticipating deterioration, optimizes internal flow, protects vulnerable patients, and ensures coherence across pathways. Coding risk gives stability and transparency to choices, helping avoid both dangerous delays and inappropriate resource use.

In short, risk stratification and triage are not separate actions but two faces of the same cognitive process: predicting and deciding. Triage operationalizes stratification; stratification gives clinical meaning to triage. Without the former, priority cannot be justified; without the latter, prediction remains abstract. In this interdependence lies the strength of the modern emergency system, built on the ability to anticipate a patient's clinical future amid uncertainty and pressure.

2.5   The Evolution of Stratification in Emergency Medicine: The Five Levels of Triage

Historically, risk stratification arose as an epidemiological and managerial need. It served to classify patients into homogeneous severity groups to compare outcomes and allocate resources. Over time, however, it became a clinical paradigm, a lens through which to read the complexity of emergency care. In the 1990s, the spread of prognostic models and severity scores in ICUs and EDs showed that quantitative risk prediction improved the consistency and safety of decisions [35, 36]. Emergency medicine, more than other fields, made such prediction a daily necessity because its mission is not only to stabilize but also, based on risk prediction, to choose pathways [35]. The progressive adoption of five-level triage systems marked a qualitative leap in this direction [20, 32, 33]. It was not merely an increase in categories but the introduction of a finer scale of risk gradation. Five levels better represent the continuum from low to high urgency, allow resource modulation, reduce overload risk, and prevent small clinical changes from causing crude jumps in priority [20, 32, 33].

More recent studies show that moving from a four- to a five-level triage system yields measurable benefits in validity, accuracy, and ED flow management [20, 32, 33]. Additional work indicates that five-level systems provide more refined discrimination for patients of moderate to high severity thanks to the added level, which allows more nuanced gradation than four broader classes [20, 32, 33]. Moreover, in overcrowded, high-volume settings, the greater granularity of five levels appears to help reduce waiting times and improve the match between resources and actual need, though gains vary by training, organization, and context [20, 32, 33]. At the same time, the literature notes that adopting a five-level system requires investment in training and procedures: without adequate support, more levels can introduce operational complexity or inconsistency in code assignment [20, 32, 33].

2.6 Practical and Educational Implications

The implications of risk stratification go beyond the decision moment to shape training and organizational culture. For stratification to work, the clinical community must accept probability as the natural language of care. That means educating professionals not only to recognize signs of severity but also to think in terms of distributions, uncertainty, and updatable forecasts. It is a paradigm shift that demands practice and reflection, not mere protocol application. Triage tools, when used well, support and sharpen intuition and make reasoning explicit, but they cannot replace clinical judgment [27, 28]. The educational challenge is to teach their intelligent use, acknowledging that stratification is first and foremost a way of thinking [27, 28]. Organizationally, embracing the logic of stratification means revisiting flows, roles, and decision thresholds. It means accepting that not all patients require the same monitoring intensity and that safety is measured not only by waiting times but also by risk prevented. It means equipping staff with rapid, reliable, reproducible instruments for estimating risk while also creating spaces to discuss and reassess cases, continually updating the collective risk map [14, 27, 28, 37, 38]. In the most advanced emergency services, stratification has become a shared language, a way to anticipate problems and reduce reliance on isolated signals by promoting a systemic reading of vulnerability.

Today, risk stratification is the keystone of emergency medicine. It is the principle that unites triage logic with clinical forecasting, organizational necessity with the ethics of priority, and the science of probability with the practice of judgment. It is at once a method and a mindset, a competency and a culture. Its strength lies in its ability to join evidence and experience, numbers and narrative, and predictability and surprise. For the emergency medicine of the future, the challenge will be to keep refining this capacity, integrating ever richer data without losing the human dimension of judgment. To stratify risk does not mean reducing the patient to a probability; it means recognizing, behind each unique story, the regularities that allow many to be saved. In this balance between science and prudence, between algorithm and intuition, triage finds its firmest footing and emergency medicine its deepest meaning.

References

1. Jaffe TA, Wang D, Loveless B, Lai D, Loesche M, White B, Raja AS, He S. A scoping review of emergency department discharge risk stratification. West J Emerg Med. 2021;22(6):1218–26. https://doi.org/10.5811/westjem.2021.6.52969. PMID: 34787544; PMCID: PMC8597698.

2. Rente MJB, Mota LAND, João ALDS. Predictive model for managing the clinical risk of emergency department patients: a systematic review. J Clin Med. 2025;14(20):7245. https://doi.org/10.3390/jcm14207245. PMID: 41156117; PMCID: PMC12565041.

3. Brabrand M, Folkestad L, Clausen NG, Knudsen T, Hallas J. Risk scoring systems for adults admitted to the emergency department: a systematic review. Scand J Trauma Resusc Emerg Med. 2010;18:8. https://doi.org/10.1186/1757-7241-18-8. PMID: 20146829; PMCID: PMC2835641.

4. Henriksen DP, Brabrand M, Lassen AT. Prognosis and risk factors for deterioration in patients admitted to a medical emergency department. PLoS One. 2014;9(4):e94649. https://doi.org/10.1371/journal.pone.0094649. PMID: 24718637; PMCID: PMC3981818.

5. Loddo S, Costaggiu D, Palimodde A, et al. Emergency department: risk stratification in the elderly. J Gerontol Geriatr. 2021;69(3):164–70. https://doi.org/10.36150/2499-6564-N352.

6. Zachariasse JM, van der Hagen V, Seiger N, Mackway-Jones K, van Veen M, Moll HA. Performance of triage systems in emergency care: a systematic review and meta-analysis. BMJ Open. 2019;9(5):e026471. https://doi.org/10.1136/bmjopen-2018-026471. PMID: 31142524; PMCID: PMC6549628.

7. Hinson JS, Martinez DA, Cabral S, George K, Whalen M, Hansoti B, Levin S. Triage performance in emergency medicine: a systematic review. Ann Emerg Med. 2019;74(1):140–52. https://doi.org/10.1016/j.annemergmed.2018.09.022. Epub 2018 Nov 22. PMID: 30470513.

8. Health Economics Unit. Risk stratification: a 'how to' guide. Birmingham: NHS; 2024.

9. Risk stratification – an overview. In: ScienceDirect Topics [Internet]. Elsevier; 2020 [cited 2025 Dec 3].

10. Yu T, Vollenweider D, Varadhan R, Li T, Boyd C, Puhan MA. Support of personalized medicine through risk-stratified treatment recommendations – an environmental scan of clinical practice guidelines. BMC Med. 2013;11:7. https://doi.org/10.1186/1741-7015-11-7. PMID: 23302096; PMCID: PMC3565912.

11. Zaboli A, Sibilio S, Massar M, Brigiari G, Magnarelli G, Parodi M, Mian M, Pfeifer N, Brigo F, Turcato G. Enhancing triage accuracy: the influence of nursing education on risk prediction. Int Emerg Nurs. 2024;75:101486. https://doi.org/10.1016/j.ienj.2024.101486. Epub 2024 Jun 26. PMID: 38936274.

12. Geary U, Kennedy U. Clinical decision-making in emergency medicine. Emergencias. 2010;22(1):56–60.

13. Marewski JN, Gigerenzer G. Heuristic decision making in medicine. Dialogues Clin Neurosci. 2012;14(1):77–89. https://doi.org/10.31887/DCNS.2012.14.1/jmarewski. PMID: 22577307; PMCID: PMC3341653.

14. Ausserhofer D, Zaboli A, Pfeifer N, Solazzo P, Magnarelli G, Marsoner T, Siller M, Turcato G. Errors in nurse-led triage: an observational study. Int J Nurs Stud. 2021;113:103788. https://doi.org/10.1016/j.ijnurstu.2020.103788. Epub 2020 Oct 8. PMID: 33120136.

15. Vainieri M, Panero C, Coletta L. Waiting times in emergency departments: a resource allocation or an efficiency issue? BMC Health Serv Res. 2020;20(1):549. https://doi.org/10.1186/s12913-020-05417-w. PMID: 32552829; PMCID: PMC7298831.

16. Horvath S, Visekruna S, Kilpatrick K, McCallum M, Carter N. Models of care with advanced practice nurses in the emergency department: a scoping review. Int J Nurs Stud. 2023;148:104608. https://doi.org/10.1016/j.ijnurstu.2023.104608. Epub 2023 Sep 18. PMID: 37801938.

17. Aacharya RP, Gastmans C, Denier Y. Emergency department triage: an ethical analysis. BMC Emerg Med. 2011;11:16. https://doi.org/10.1186/1471-227X-11-16. PMID: 21982119; PMCID: PMC3199257.

18. Moskop JC, Iserson KV. Triage in medicine, part II: underlying values and principles. Ann Emerg Med. 2007;49(3):282–7. https://doi.org/10.1016/j.annemergmed.2006.07.012. Epub 2006 Aug 14. PMID: 17141137.
19. Liu T, Gu Y, Chen H, Zhang Y, Zheng L, Huang X, Xu Y, Wen C, Chen M, Lin J, Huang D, Chen F, Zhong Y, Chen H, Guo Y, Lu M, Zhang G, Wu H, Wang C, Xi X, Li L, Yu T. A foundational triage system for improving accuracy in moderate acuity level emergency classifications. Commun Med (Lond). 2025;5(1):322. https://doi.org/10.1038/s43856-025-01052-w. PMID: 40745473; PMCID: PMC12314101.
20. Kuriyama A, Urushidani S, Nakayama T. Five-level emergency triage systems: variation in assessment of validity. Emerg Med J. 2017;34(11):703–10. https://doi.org/10.1136/emermed-2016-206295. Epub 2017 Jul 27. PMID: 28751363.
21. Oh WO, Jung MJ. Triage-clinical reasoning on emergency nursing competency: a multiple linear mediation effect. BMC Nurs. 2024;23(1):274. https://doi.org/10.1186/s12912-024-01919-8. PMID: 38658947; PMCID: PMC11044571.
22. Royal College of Emergency Medicine. CC5: Decision making and clinical reasoning. In: Curriculum for training in emergency medicine. London: RCEM; 2021.
23. Egoda Kapuralalage TN, Chan HF, Dulleck U, Hughes JA, Torgler B, Whyte S. Clinical decision-making: cognitive biases and heuristics in triage decisions in the emergency department. Am J Emerg Med. 2025;92:60–7. https://doi.org/10.1016/j.ajem.2025.02.043. Epub 2025 Feb 27. PMID: 40073709.
24. Cioffi J. Decision making by emergency nurses in triage assessments. Accid Emerg Nurs. 1998;6(4):184–91. https://doi.org/10.1016/s0965-2302(98)90077-7. PMID: 10232095.
25. Lorenzini G, Zamboni A, Gelati L, Di Martino A, Pellacani A, Barbieri N, Baraldi M. Emergency team competencies: scoping review for the development of a tool to support the briefing and debriefing activities of emergency healthcare providers. J Anesth Analg Crit Care. 2023;3(1):24. https://doi.org/10.1186/s44158-023-00109-3. PMID: 37507807; PMCID: PMC10386683.
26. Gilboy N, Tanabe T, Travers D, Rosenau AM. Emergency Severity Index (ESI): a triage tool for emergency department care. Version 4. In: Implementation handbook, AHRQ Publication No. 05-0046-2. Rockville: Agency for Healthcare Research and Quality; 2005.
27. Manchester Triage Group. Emergency triage. 2nd ed. Malden: Blackwell Publishing; 2006. https://doi.org/10.1002/9780470757321.
28. Robertson-Steel I. Evolution of triage systems. Emerg Med J. 2006;23(2):154–5. https://doi.org/10.1136/emj.2005.030270. PMID: 16439754; PMCID: PMC2564046.
29. Kutz A, Hausfater P, Amin D, Amin A, Canavaggio P, Sauvin G, Bernard M, Conca A, Haubitz S, Struja T, Huber A, Mueller B, Schuetz P, TRIAGE study group. The TRIAGE-ProADM score for an early risk stratification of medical patients in the emergency department – development based on a multi-national, prospective, observational study. PLoS One. 2016;11(12):e0168076. https://doi.org/10.1371/journal.pone.0168076. PMID: 28005916; PMCID: PMC5179054.
30. Challen K. How good is triage, and what is it good for? Emerg Med J. 2017;34(11):702. https://doi.org/10.1136/emermed-2017-206973. Epub 2017 Oct 4. PMID: 28978651.
31. Zaboli A. Establishing a common ground: the future of triage systems. BMC Emerg Med. 2024;24(1):148. https://doi.org/10.1186/s12873-024-01070-2. PMID: 39148042; PMCID: PMC11328465.
32. Kongensgaard FT, Fløjstrup M, Lassen A, Dahlin J, Brabrand M. Are 5-level triage systems improved by using a symptom based approach?-a Danish cohort study. Scand J Trauma Resusc Emerg Med. 2022;30(1):31. https://doi.org/10.1186/s13049-022-01016-2. PMID: 35468799; PMCID: PMC9036764.
33. Travers DA, Waller AE, Bowling JM, Flowers D, Tintinalli J. Five-level triage system more effective than three-level in tertiary emergency department. J Emerg Nurs. 2002;28(5):395–400. https://doi.org/10.1067/men.2002.127184. PMID: 12386619.

34. Peta D, Day A, Lugari WS, Gorman V, Ahayalimudin N, Pajo VMT. Triage: a global perspective. J Emerg Nurs. 2023;49(6):814–25. https://doi.org/10.1016/j.jen.2023.08.004. PMID: 37925222.
35. Chan SL, Lee JW, Ong MEH, Siddiqui FJ, Graves N, Ho AFW, Liu N. Implementation of prediction models in the emergency department from an implementation science perspective-determinants, outcomes, and real-world impact: a scoping review. Ann Emerg Med. 2023;82(1):22–36. https://doi.org/10.1016/j.annemergmed.2023.02.001. Epub 2023 Mar 14. PMID: 36925394.
36. Lapp L, Roper M, Kavanagh K, Bouamrane MM, Schraag S. Dynamic prediction of patient outcomes in the intensive Care unit: a scoping review of the state-of-the-art. J Intensive Care Med. 2023;38(7):575–91. https://doi.org/10.1177/08850666231166349. Epub 2023 Apr 5. PMID: 37016893; PMCID: PMC10302367
37. Zaboli A, Sibilio S, Magnarelli G, Rella E, Fanni Canelles M, Pfeifer N, Brigo F, Turcato G. Daily triage audit can improve nurses' triage stratification: a pre-post study. J Adv Nurs. 2023;79(2):605–15. https://doi.org/10.1111/jan.15521. Epub 2022 Dec 1. PMID: 36453458.
38. Zaboli A, Battisti D, Ziller M, Turcato G, Camporesi S. Can patients' characteristics influence triage errors? A Quasi-Experimental study. Int Emerg Nurs. 2025;81:101647. https://doi.org/10.1016/j.ienj.2025.101647. Epub 2025 Jun 28. PMID: 40580650.

The Healthcare Professional and Triage 3

Triage represents one of the most critical and complex clinical functions within emergency medicine, requiring a unique synthesis of technical competencies, decision-making capacity, communication skills, and the management of clinical risk under extreme time pressure [1, 2]. Defining the most appropriate professional profile for this function has been the subject of scientific and organizational debate that has traversed various evolutionary phases, from the initial, predominantly physician-centered conception to the current recognition of the specialized nursing role as the international reference standard. The strategic importance of this professional choice transcends purely operational aspects, encompassing patient safety, economic sustainability, organizational efficiency, and quality of care. The scientific literature of the past three decades has provided consistent evidence supporting not only the appropriateness of the nursing role in triage but also the necessity of structured approaches to training, maintenance of competencies, and the management of the multiple factors that influence decision quality in this specific clinical context [3–5].

3.1 Foundations of the Professional Choice: From the Physician–Nurse Debate to International Consensus

The debate on the most appropriate professional figure for triage characterized the 1970s and 1990s, when the systematic implementation of these processes in civilian emergency departments required clear definitions of roles and responsibilities [6, 7]. The initial arguments in favor of physician involvement were based on the complexity of decision-making and the clinical/legal responsibility inherent in prioritization decisions [7]. However, outcome studies and the assessment of operational sustainability progressively favored the nursing model [6, 7]. A study by Considine et al. (2000) demonstrated that nurse triage, when supported by structured training

© The Author(s), under exclusive license to Springer Nature Switzerland AG 2026

A. Zaboli, G. Turcato, *Triage Systems: Essential Knowledge for Emergency Nurses and Physicians*, https://doi.org/10.1007/978-3-032-20825-5_3

and standardized protocols, achieved good accuracy levels, with significant advantages in operational costs and organizational sustainability [8]. More recently, a systematic review and meta-analysis of advanced nurse-led triage protocols found that such protocols reduce emergency department length of stay without compromising safety and are associated with higher patient and staff satisfaction, reinforcing the central role of nurses in delivering effective and efficient triage [9].

The success of the nursing model in triage rests on a specific set of competencies that characterize the nursing profession and are particularly well suited to the demands of this process: holistic assessment and rapid assessment. Nurses are trained for a holistic appraisal that integrates physiological parameters, clinical observation, targeted history-taking, and psychosocial evaluation into an overall risk framework [10, 11]. This competence, developed through foundational training and consolidated in clinical practice, translates into pattern-recognition capabilities that enable the rapid identification of warning signs even in atypical presentations [10, 11].

Nursing education emphasizes clinical risk management and the ability to make appropriate decisions under conditions of informational uncertainty. These competencies transfer directly to the triage context, where the objective is not definitive diagnosis but the accurate estimation of immediate risk and temporal priority [12].

Educational research in triage has identified specific components that must characterize initial training programs to ensure appropriate competencies and clinical safety: structured theoretical training [12]. Research in triage has shown that structured educational programs, combining theoretical instruction on emergency pathophysiology, the principles of the adopted triage system, risk management, and communication in emergencies with scenario-based practice, significantly improve triage nurses' decision-making skills and the accuracy of prioritization compared with informal on-the-job learning [13, 14].

Finally, a period of preceptorship is a critical element in the transition from theory to practice [1]. Guidelines from the International Association for Healthcare Quality recommend a minimum of 40 h of supervised preceptorship with structured feedback, based on specific competency checklists and the progressive assessment of decision-making autonomy [15].

Studies have documented that triage competencies, if not constantly practiced and updated, tend to deteriorate over time [16]. This phenomenon, known as "skill decay," represents a critical challenge for the quality and safety of the process [16]. A recent study on triage education has shown that the benefits of initial training may diminish within a few months in the absence of structured refresher programs. In a quasi-experimental study of 117 nurses, Pontisidis et al. reported that a triage education program using both the Emergency Severity Index and the Australian Triage Scale produced significant improvements in triage knowledge, skills, and accuracy immediately after training, but that these gains had partially declined at three-month follow-up, underscoring the need for ongoing education [17].

A recent scoping review of refresher training for emergency department triage nurses corroborates these findings, concluding that periodic retraining is necessary to maintain triage accuracy and counteract skill decay over time [18].

The literature has identified specific strategies effective for maintaining competencies:

- Structured Periodic Updates: Sessions focused on red flags, special populations, and evidence-based updates have proven effective in maintaining stable accuracy levels over time [12–14].
- Audit and Individualized Feedback: Programs of systematic audit of triage decisions with personalized feedback improve concordance with standards and reduce inter-operator variability [1, 19].

3.2   Defining the Triage Nurse

The triage nurse represents a specialized professional figure within emergency nursing, characterized by a unique combination of clinical competencies, decision-making capabilities, communication skills, and stress management abilities that distinguish this role from other nursing functions. The triage nurse operates primarily as a clinical decision-maker and risk assessor, functioning at the critical interface between the undifferentiated patient population seeking emergency care and the structured resources of the Emergency Department.

International professional guidance from nursing and emergency medicine organizations describes triage as an advanced nursing role. Documents from the Emergency Nurses Association and the National Emergency Nurses Association, together with the Australasian College for Emergency Medicine guidelines on the Australasian Triage Scale, specify that triage should be performed by registered nurses with emergency experience and triage-specific education [20–22]. These nurses are responsible for the rapid initial assessment of all patients presenting to the Emergency Department, the assignment of a priority level using validated five-level triage systems, the initiation of selected protocol-driven interventions when indicated, and the ongoing observation and reassessment of patients while they await definitive medical evaluation [20–22].

The scientific literature and international guidelines have progressively defined minimum prerequisites for assuming the triage role, moving from informal approaches based primarily on seniority toward competency-based selection models.

Clinical Experience: A minimum of 12–24 months of emergency department experience is considered essential to develop the pattern recognition capabilities and clinical judgment necessary for rapid risk assessment [1, 15, 20–22].

Foundational Competencies: Proficiency in physical assessment, interpretation of vital signs in clinical context, and recognition of danger signs across major body systems represent non-negotiable prerequisites [1, 15, 20–22].

Communication and Interpersonal Skills: The ability to rapidly establish rapport, elicit focused history from distressed or uncooperative patients, communicate effectively with diverse populations (linguistic, cultural, and age-related), and manage conflict situations represents a critical competency domain [1, 15, 20–22].

The organizational positioning of the triage nurse varies across international models, but contemporary best practices converge on several key principles. The triage nurse typically operates with a high degree of autonomy within defined protocols [20–22].

3.3 The Temporal Architecture of Triage Assessment

The triage encounter represents a highly structured clinical interaction characterized by extreme temporal compression. International guidelines specify target assessment times ranging from 2 to 5 min per patient, creating a unique clinical paradigm where comprehensive assessment must be sacrificed in favor of focused risk evaluation [15, 22]. Understanding the temporal architecture of this process is essential to appreciate both its capabilities and limitations.

The Sequential Phases of Triage Assessment:

Phase 1—Across-the-Room Assessment: The triage encounter begins before verbal interaction, with what experienced nurses describe as the "across-the-room assessment" or "general impression." This initial visual evaluation assesses work of breathing (respiratory rate, use of accessory muscles, nasal flaring, positioning, audible stridor, or wheezing); perfusion status (skin color, diaphoresis, and capillary refill); neurological status (level of consciousness, appropriateness of interaction, speech clarity, and facial expressions provide initial neurological screening); pain and distress (facial expressions, body positioning, vocalizations, and protective behaviors indicate pain severity and location); and mobility and functional status (the patient's ability to ambulate, self-position, and perform basic movements) [1, 15, 23].

Phase 2—Chief Complaint and Focused History: following the initial visual assessment, the triage nurse elicits the chief complaint and obtains focused historical information. This phase differs fundamentally from comprehensive history-taking, employing structured questioning strategies designed to maximize information yield within severe time constraints [1, 15, 23]. The opening question typically follows the format "What brought you to the Emergency Department today?" the former elicits the patient's primary concern, while the latter may generate unfocused narratives.

Phase 3—Vital Signs Measurement and Interpretation: vital signs represent the objective foundation of triage assessment, providing quantifiable physiological data that must be interpreted within clinical context [1, 15, 23]. Raw vital sign values must be interpreted within clinical context. A heart rate of 110 bpm may represent normal physiological response to pain or anxiety in a young adult, compensatory tachycardia in early shock, or primary cardiac dysrhythmia. The triage nurse's clinical judgment distinguishes these scenarios through integration with other assessment components.

Phase 4—Focused Physical Examination: The triage physical examination differs fundamentally from the comprehensive examination, focusing exclusively on assessment elements that inform priority decisions. This examination is guided by the chief complaint and initial assessment findings.

Certain physical examination findings mandate immediate priority escalation regardless of other assessment components, for example, unresponsiveness or profound altered mental status (GCS ≤ 8), or absent or agonal respirations, absent central pulses, or active uncontrolled hemorrhage, or signs of impending airway compromise.

Phase 5—Priority Assignment and Documentation: Following assessment completion, the triage nurse assigns a priority level according to the implemented triage system. This decision integrates all assessment components—visual impression, history, vital signs, and physical examination—within the structured framework of the triage algorithm. Modern triage systems employ algorithmic approaches that guide priority assignment [1, 15, 20, 22]. Triage documentation must capture essential assessment elements while maintaining efficiency.

Phase 6—Initiation of Care and Patient Disposition: The final phase of triage involves initiation of appropriate interventions within standing orders, patient education regarding expected waiting times, and physical disposition to the appropriate waiting area.

3.4 Continuous Monitoring and Re-triage

The triage nurse's responsibility extends beyond initial assessment to include continuous monitoring of patients in the waiting area. International guidelines specify maximum waiting times, which depend on the triage systems, before mandatory re-assessment [1, 15, 20, 22].

3.5 The Professional at the Core: Balancing Clinical Judgment and Standardization in Triage

Triage is one of the most critical and complex decision-making processes in emergency medicine, defined by the need to make accurate clinical judgments under intense time pressure, with incomplete information and limited resources [1, 20, 22]. In this context, the ability to quickly distinguish between patients who need immediate intervention and those who can safely wait is vitally important, not only for individual clinical outcomes but also for the efficiency and sustainability of the entire health system. The contemporary relevance of triage is measured primarily by its evolution from a predominantly intuitive, subjective process into a structured, objective system grounded in scientific evidence [24, 25]. This transformation is not merely methodological; it is a necessary response to rising demands for patient safety, equity of access to care, transparent decisions, and professional accountability that characterize modern health systems [26, 27].

The scientific literature has consistently documented the limitations of triage systems based largely on subjective judgment [25, 27]. Studies conducted on traditional three-level priority systems have shown inter-rater reliability coefficients (kappa) frequently below 0.60, the threshold usually considered the minimum acceptable for clinical concordance [28, 29]. Cognitive psychology research applied to emergency medicine has identified numerous systematic biases that affect subjective triage decision-making [30]. Anchoring bias, where the first clinical impression disproportionately shapes subsequent judgments, was documented in high rate of triage decisions in an observational study [30–32]. Particularly concerning are findings on demographic and social bias. Some studies reported that Black/African-American patients received lower priority codes than white patients with identical clinical presentations [33–35]. Likewise, older patients were underestimated compared with younger patients with comparable clinical features [36, 37].

Subjectivity in triage is further amplified by environmental and organizational factors [38–40]. Studies documented significant variation in triage accuracy related to departmental workload: during peak influxes, prioritization accuracy fell significantly, with proportional increases in both under- and over-triage [38–40].

The shift from traditional three-level systems to structured five-level scales represents an evidence-based response to the documented limits of subjectivity [41–43]. The Emergency Severity Index, the Manchester Triage System, the Canadian Triage and Acuity Scale, the Australasian Triage Scale, and the South African Triage Scale share methodological principles that significantly reduce inter-rater variability [41–45]. Multiple studies have shown that adopting five-level systems improves kappa and reduces inter-operator variation [41–45].

Modern triage systems use standardized descriptors of clinical presentation that link observed symptoms and signs to predefined priority levels [24, 25]. The Manchester Triage System, for example, employs 52 flowcharts that guide the clinician through specific clinical discriminators, thereby reducing interpretive subjectivity [1]. Integrating objective vital-sign parameters is a fundamental pillar of objectification. "Danger-zone vital signs" define specific physiological thresholds that automatically trigger higher priority levels. The Emergency Severity Index uses vital-sign thresholds as mandatory modifiers of priority [15]. Objective pain assessment via validated numerical scales (NRS 0–10) or behavioral scales for non-communicative patients is another key element [1]. Objectifying triage also enables continuous quality monitoring through specific quantitative indicators, and it has been shown to improve patient safety by reducing prioritization errors [46, 47].

3.6   Integration Between Standardization and Personalization

Objectifying triage does not mean eliminating clinical judgment but structuring it within evidence-based frameworks that enhance its effectiveness while reducing inappropriate variability [48, 49]. Some studies have shown that experienced nurses use clinical overrides effectively in a meaningful proportion of cases, thereby increasing accuracy [49, 50]. This underscores the importance of preserving space for professional judgment within structured systems. Triage necessarily operates amid diagnostic uncertainty, where the goal is not to make definitive diagnoses but to estimate immediate clinical risk. In this setting, expert clinical judgment remains irreplaceable for interpreting weak signals, contextual information, and atypical patterns that may escape standardized criteria [49].

Implementing scheduled re-evaluation triggers is a key mechanism for managing uncertainty: patients initially classified as non-urgent are systematically reassessed at predefined intervals, allowing clinicians to detect clinical deterioration or unexpected evolution [1, 15, 22]. Structured training programs that combine mastery of standardized criteria with the development of clinical competencies have proven effective in improving both the accuracy and the consistency of triage decisions [17, 18].

Thus, the evolution of triage from subjectivity toward objectification is a foundational paradigm of contemporary emergency medicine, mirroring broader shifts toward evidence-based practice, structured quality systems, and professional accountability [24, 25]. The evidence clearly shows that using objective, standardized, auditable criteria significantly improves patient safety, equity of access, and organizational efficiency [25, 48]. However, objectification should not be understood as mechanizing the clinical process but as structuring professional judgment within evidence-based frameworks that amplify its effectiveness while curbing inappropriate variability. Triage remains, at its core, a clinical process requiring skills, experience, and management of uncertainty that cannot be fully reduced to algorithms. The ultimate aim remains unchanged from triage's historical origins: identify those who cannot wait and ensure that limited resources are allocated to maximize benefit for the greatest number, using tools, methods, and quality safeguards that reflect the highest standards of modern medicine.

The relevance of triage is therefore measured by its ability to combine scientific rigor with the humanity of care, objectified processes with personalized interventions, and organizational efficiency with patient-centeredness. From this perspective, objectification is not an endpoint but an evolutionary stage toward ever more sophisticated, safe, and effective triage systems that keep at their center the fundamental mission of protecting human life when time is the most precious resource.

References

1. Mackway-Jones K, Marsden J, Windle J. Emergency triage: Manchester triage group. 3rd ed. Oxford: Wiley-Blackwell; 2014.
2. Christ M, Grossmann F, Winter D, Bingisser R, Platz E. Modern triage in the emergency department. Dtsch Arztebl Int. 2010;107(50):892–8. https://doi.org/10.3238/arztebl.2010.0892. Epub 2010 Dec 17
3. Considine J, Botti M, Thomas S. Do knowledge and experience have specific roles in triage decision-making? Acad Emerg Med. 2007;14(8):722–6. https://doi.org/10.1197/j.aem.2007.04.015.
4. Yu M, Ma L, Ma Q. Competency of triage nurse in the emergency department: a scoping review protocol. PLoS One. 2025;20(9):e0331982. https://doi.org/10.1371/journal.pone.0331982.
5. Oh WO, Jung MJ. Triage-clinical reasoning on emergency nursing competency: a multiple linear mediation effect. BMC Nurs. 2024;23(1):274. https://doi.org/10.1186/s12912-024-01919-8.

6. Mills J, Webster AL, Wofsy CB, Harding P, D'Acuti D. Effectiveness of nurse triage in the emergency department of an urban county hospital. JACEP. 1976;5(11):877–82. https://doi.org/10.1016/s0361-1124(76)80034-2.

7. De Angelis C, McHugh M. The effectiveness of various health personnel as triage agents. J Community Health. 1977;2(4):268–77. https://doi.org/10.1007/BF01325148.

8. Considine J, Ung L, Thomas S. Triage nurses' decisions using the National Triage Scale for Australian emergency departments. Accid Emerg Nurs. 2000;8(4):201–9. https://doi.org/10.1054/aaen.2000.0166.

9. Soster CB, Anschau F, Rodrigues NH, Silva LGAD, Klafke A. Advanced triage protocols in the emergency department: a systematic review and meta-analysis. Rev Lat Am Enfermagem. 2022;30:e3511. https://doi.org/10.1590/1518-8345.5479.3511.

10. Gorick H, McGee M, Wilson G, Williams E, Patel J, Zonato A, Ayodele W, Shams S, Di Battista L, Smith TO. Understanding triage assessment of acuity by emergency nurses at initial adult patient presentation: a qualitative systematic review. Int Emerg Nurs. 2023;71:101334. https://doi.org/10.1016/j.ienj.2023.101334. Epub 2023 Sep 14

11. Gorick H, McGee M, Smith TO. Assessments under pressure: interviews with triage nurses in emergency departments: an exploratory descriptive qualitative study. J Adv Nurs. 2025; https://doi.org/10.1111/jan.70283. Epub ahead of print

12. Zaboli A, Sibilio S, Massar M, Brigiari G, Magnarelli G, Parodi M, Mian M, Pfeifer N, Brigo F, Turcato G. Enhancing triage accuracy: the influence of nursing education on risk prediction. Int Emerg Nurs. 2024;75:101486. https://doi.org/10.1016/j.ienj.2024.101486. Epub 2024 Jun 26

13. Recznik CT, Simko LC, Travers D, Devido J. Pediatric triage education for the general emergency nurse: a randomized crossover trial comparing simulation with paper-case studies. J Emerg Nurs. 2019;45(4):394–402. https://doi.org/10.1016/j.jen.2019.01.009. Epub 2019 Mar 1

14. Wolf L. Does your staff really "get" initial patient assessment? Assessing competency in triage using simulated patient encounters. J Emerg Nurs. 2010;36(4):370–4. https://doi.org/10.1016/j.jen.2010.04.016. Epub 2010 May 31

15. Gilboy N, Tanabe P, Travers DA, Rosenau AM, Eitel DR. Emergency severity index (ESI), version 4: implementation handbook. Rockville (MD): Agency for Healthcare Research and Quality (US); 2005. (AHRQ Publication No. 05-0046-2)

16. Brosinski CM, Riddell AJ, Valdez S. Improving triage accuracy: a staff development approach. Clin Nurse Spec. 2017;31(3):145–8. https://doi.org/10.1097/NUR.0000000000000291.

17. Pontisidis G, Bellali T, Galanis P, Polyzos N. Effect of triage training on nurses with emergency severity index and Australian triage scale: a quasi-experimental study. AIMS Public Health. 2024;11(4):1049–70. https://doi.org/10.3934/publichealth.2024054.

18. Hinds A, Kay S, Evans K. Refresher training for emergency department triage nurses - a scoping review. Australas Emerg Care. 2025;28(3):204–12. https://doi.org/10.1016/j.auec.2025.03.006. Epub 2025 Apr 16

19. Zaboli A, Sibilio S, Magnarelli G, Rella E, Fanni Canelles M, Pfeifer N, Brigo F, Turcato G. Daily triage audit can improve nurses' triage stratification: a pre-post study. J Adv Nurs. 2023;79(2):605–15. https://doi.org/10.1111/jan.15521. Epub 2022 Dec 1

20. Emergency Nurses Association. Triage qualifications and competency. J Emerg Nurs. 2017;43(6):571–4.

21. National Emergency Nurses Association. Position statement: role of the triage nurse. Chilliwack (BC): National Emergency Nurses Association; 2019.

22. Australasian College for Emergency Medicine. Guidelines on the implementation of the Australasian triage scale in emergency departments. Melbourne: Australasian College for Emergency Medicine; 2016.

23. Canadian Association of Emergency Physicians; National Emergency Nurses Affiliation; et al. The Canadian Triage and Acuity Scale (CTAS)—participant manual v2.5b. Ottawa; 2013.

24. Hinson JS, Martinez DA, Cabral S, et al. Triage performance in emergency medicine: a systematic review. Ann Emerg Med. 2019;74(1):140–52. https://doi.org/10.1016/j.annemergmed.2018.09.022.

25. Zachariasse JM, van der Hagen V, Seiger N, Mackway-Jones K, van Veen M, Moll HA. Performance of triage systems in emergency care: a systematic review and meta-analysis. BMJ Open. 2019;9(5):e026471. Published 2019 May 28. https://doi.org/10.1136/bmjopen-2018-026471.

26. Moll HA. Challenges in the validation of triage systems at emergency departments. J Clin Epidemiol. 2010;63(4):384–8. https://doi.org/10.1016/j.jclinepi.2009.07.009.

27. Kuriyama A, Urushidani S, Nakayama T. Five-level emergency triage systems: variation in assessment of validity. Emerg Med J. 2017;34(11):703–10. https://doi.org/10.1136/emermed-2016-206295.

28. van der Wulp I, van Stel HF. Calculating kappas from adjusted data improved the comparability of the reliability of triage systems: a comparative study. J Clin Epidemiol. 2010;63(11):1256–63. https://doi.org/10.1016/j.jclinepi.2010.01.012.

29. van der Wulp I, van Stel HF. Adjusting weighted kappa for severity of mistriage decreases reported reliability of emergency department triage systems: a comparative study. J Clin Epidemiol. 2009;62(11):1196–201. https://doi.org/10.1016/j.jclinepi.2009.01.007.

30. Egoda Kapuralalage TN, Chan HF, Dulleck U, Hughes JA, Torgler B, Whyte S. Clinical decision-making: cognitive biases and heuristics in triage decisions in the emergency department. Am J Emerg Med. 2025;92:60–7. https://doi.org/10.1016/j.ajem.2025.02.043.

31. Dargahi H, Monajemi A, Soltani A, Nejad Nedaie HH, Labaf A. Anchoring errors in emergency medicine residents and faculties. Med J Islam Repub Iran. 2022;36:124. Published 2022 Oct 26. https://doi.org/10.47176/mjiri.36.124.

32. Daniel M, Khandelwal S, Santen SA, Malone M, Croskerry P. Cognitive debiasing strategies for the emergency department. AEM Educ Train. 2017;1(1):41–2. Published 2017 Jan 19. https://doi.org/10.1002/aet2.10010.

33. Schrader CD, Lewis LM. Racial disparity in emergency department triage. J Emerg Med. 2013;44(2):511–8. https://doi.org/10.1016/j.jemermed.2012.05.010.

34. Peitzman C, Carreras Tartak JA, Samuels-Kalow M, Raja A, Macias-Konstantopoulos WL. Racial differences in triage for emergency department patients with subjective chief complaints. West J Emerg Med. 2023;24(5):888–93. https://doi.org/10.5811/westjem.59044.

35. Joseph JW, Kennedy M, Landry AM, et al. Race and ethnicity and primary language in emergency department triage. JAMA Netw Open. 2023;6(10):e2337557. Published 2023 Oct 2. https://doi.org/10.1001/jamanetworkopen.2023.37557.

36. Ginsburg AD, Oliveira JE, Silva L, Mullan A, et al. Should age be incorporated into the adult triage algorithm in the emergency department? Am J Emerg Med. 2021;46:508–14. https://doi.org/10.1016/j.ajem.2020.10.075.

37. Grossmann FF, Zumbrunn T, Frauchiger A, Delport K, Bingisser R, Nickel CH. At risk of undertriage? Testing the performance and accuracy of the emergency severity index in older emergency department patients. Ann Emerg Med. 2012;60(3):317–25.e3. https://doi.org/10.1016/j.annemergmed.2011.12.013.

38. Morley C, Unwin M, Peterson GM, Stankovich J, Kinsman L. Emergency department crowding: a systematic review of causes, consequences and solutions. PLoS One. 2018;13(8):e0203316. Published 2018 Aug 30. https://doi.org/10.1371/journal.pone.0203316.

39. Chen W, Linthicum B, Argon NT, et al. The effects of emergency department crowding on triage and hospital admission decisions. Am J Emerg Med. 2020;38(4):774–9. https://doi.org/10.1016/j.ajem.2019.06.039.

40. van der Linden MC, Meester BE, van der Linden N. Emergency department crowding affects triage processes. Int Emerg Nurs. 2016;29:27–31. https://doi.org/10.1016/j.ienj.2016.02.003.

41. Wuerz RC, Milne LW, Eitel DR, Travers D, Gilboy N. Reliability and validity of a new five-level triage instrument. Acad Emerg Med. 2000;7(3):236–42. https://doi.org/10.1111/j.1553-2712.2000.tb01066.

42. Beveridge R, Ducharme J, Janes L, Beaulieu S, Walter S. Reliability of the Canadian emergency department triage and acuity scale: interrater agreement. Ann Emerg Med. 1999;34(2):155–9. https://doi.org/10.1016/s0196-0644(99)70223-4.

43. Manos D, Petrie DA, Beveridge RC, Walter S, Ducharme J. Inter-observer agreement using the Canadian emergency department triage and acuity scale. CJEM. 2002;4(1):16–22. https://doi.org/10.1017/s1481803500006023.
44. Twomey M, Wallis LA, Thompson ML, Myers JE. The South African Triage Scale (adult version) provides reliable acuity ratings. Int Emerg Nurs. 2012;20(3):142–50. https://doi.org/10.1016/j.ienj.2011.08.002.
45. Azeredo TR, Guedes HM, Rebelo de Almeida RA, Chianca TC, Martins JC. Efficacy of the Manchester triage system: a systematic review. Int Emerg Nurs. 2015;23(2):47–52. https://doi.org/10.1016/j.ienj.2014.06.001.
46. Ouellet S, Galliani MC, Gélinas C, et al. Strategies to improve the quality of nurse triage in emergency departments: a realist review protocol. Nurs Open. 2023;10(5):2770–9. https://doi.org/10.1002/nop2.1550.
47. Savioli G, Ceresa IF, Gri N, et al. Emergency department overcrowding: understanding the factors to find corresponding solutions. J Pers Med. 2022;12(2):279. Published 2022 Feb 14. https://doi.org/10.3390/jpm12020279.
48. Gilboy N, Travers D, Wuerz R. Re-evaluating triage in the new millennium: a comprehensive look at the need for standardization and quality. J Emerg Nurs. 1999;25(6):468–73. https://doi.org/10.1016/s0099-1767(99)70007-3.
49. Zaboli A, Brigo F, Brigiari G, et al. Comparing safety and accuracy of standardised versus subjective triage code assignment by nurses: a multicenter observational simulated study. J Clin Nurs. 2024; https://doi.org/10.1111/jocn.17615. Online ahead of print
50. Zagalioti SC, Ziaka M, Exadaktylos A, Fyntanidou B. An effective triage education method for triage nurses: an overview and update. Open Access Emerg Med. 2025;17:105–12. Published 2025 Feb 11. https://doi.org/10.2147/OAEM.S498085.

Part II

The Current Triage Systems

Current Validated Triage System

4

This chapter introduces the principal triage systems that are currently validated and widely implemented at the international level (ATS, SATS, MTS, CTAS, and ESI) and then describes each of them in turn. Although they originated in different healthcare contexts, they share a common architecture: a five-level urgency classification, explicit criteria for clinical priority assignment, operational guidance on target waiting times, and minimum requirements for training and audit to ensure reliability over time [1–3].

In everyday practice, these scales converge on several core pillars: the structured use of clinical signs and vital parameters as urgency discriminators; the linkage of each priority level to specific time targets for initiation of assessment and treatment; and recommendations for reassessment while waiting and for monitoring quality indicators [1–3]. Expressed differently across systems and countries, these elements constitute the operational language that enables benchmarking, clinical governance, and continuous quality improvement [1, 3, 4].

The decision to focus on ATS, SATS, MTS, CTAS, and ESI is grounded both in their global diffusion and in the robustness of the available evidence [1, 2, 4].

For these reasons, this book concentrates on ATS, SATS, MTS, CTAS, and ESI as the reference triage systems. They represent the most extensively studied and widely adopted models currently available, embody the methodological shift from largely subjective three-level systems to structured five-level scales, and provide a shared framework of concepts and indicators that enables meaningful comparison of practice and outcomes across different emergency care settings [1, 2].

© The Author(s), under exclusive license to Springer Nature
Switzerland AG 2026
A. Zaboli, G. Turcato, *Triage Systems: Essential Knowledge for Emergency
Nurses and Physicians*, https://doi.org/10.1007/978-3-032-20825-5_4

4.1   Australasian Triage Scale (ATS)

4.1.1   Introduction

The ATS is the official reference triage system for ED in Australia and New Zealand. Structured into five urgency levels, the ATS orders access to care on the basis of clinical severity rather than time of arrival, with target assessment times ranging from immediate for Category 1 to a maximum of 120 minutes for Category 5 [5]. The methodological framework of the system is designed to correctly prioritize patients at higher risk of clinical deterioration or requiring time-critical treatment [5, 6].

More than a simple priority scale, the ATS represents an organizational philosophy that integrates clinical and managerial dimensions [5, 6]. Each category is not only an indicator of the urgency of the individual patient but also a service performance parameter used to monitor flow efficiency and the quality of clinical responses [5, 6]. The ATS is therefore conceived as a dual-read system: an immediate decision-making tool for the triage nurse and, at the same time, a control metric for ED governance [5–7].

Its effectiveness lies in its simplicity and standardized application. The five categories progressively reflect the degree of urgency, linking the clinical picture to realistic target times in line with the "right care, right time" philosophy [5, 6]. This linearity makes the system easy to interpret and adapt, promoting homogeneous use across hospitals of different complexity, from large metropolitan centers to small rural EDs [5–7].

A distinctive feature of the ATS is its operational immediacy. Assessment must be rapid and focused on key clinical signs and physiological stability, enabling the triage nurse to assign the most appropriate priority without resorting to complex procedures [5–7]. In this way, the ATS combines clinical rigor with decisional agility, valuing the professional judgment of the nurse within a uniform framework provided by shared and validated criteria. Adoption of the system has supported the spread, in the Australasian context, of a culture of safety and clinical accountability, with the introduction of quality indicators, regular audits, and national training programs to maintain coherence in its application [5–7]. Within this framework, the triage nurse is no longer a mere gatekeeper but an active clinical assessor, able to influence both patient outcomes and the overall efficiency of the Emergency Department.

4.1.2   History: Origin, Context of Development and Evolution

The ATS originated in Australia in the early 1990s, at a time when the public health system was facing a progressive increase in ED attendances and growing pressure on the response capacity of emergency services [5, 8]. The absence of a common language for assessing patient severity resulted in marked heterogeneity between hospitals, where each ED used its own criteria, often based on individual staff experience, with consequent significant variation in treatment times, resource use, and patient safety.

In 1993, a working group of the Australasian College for Emergency Medicine (ACEM) developed the first version of the National Triage Scale (NTS), with the aim of creating a single, reproducible system that could be applied consistently across all Australian Emergency Departments [8]. The NTS introduced, for the first time, a five-category scale, each associated with a target treatment time [8]. This approach, innovative for its time, represented a real paradigm shift. Patient assessment was no longer simply aimed at ordering access to care but at quantifying clinical risk in relation to time, establishing urgency as an objective, measurable criterion directly linked to outcomes [8].

The conceptual framework of the NTS soon proved effective and became the starting point for further methodological developments [8]. The experience accumulated over subsequent years led to the formalization of the ATS, an updated and harmonized version of the original model [8]. Official adoption by ACEM consolidated the ATS as the national standard for Australia and New Zealand, promoting its integration into information systems, educational programs and hospital protocols [5, 8, 9]. This step constituted a significant conceptual evolution. The system was refined with more specific clinical descriptors for each level, examples of typical presentations, and a clear distinction between time to assessment and time to treatment. Triage thus became not only an operational tool but also a quality and performance indicator for the emergency system, capable of measuring adherence to temporal standards and identifying organizational bottlenecks [5, 8, 9].

Further refinements were introduced to address the increasing complexity of patients [5, 8, 9]. Population aging and the growth of chronic conditions led to additional adjustments to the system and to the promotion of training tools aimed at ensuring interpretative consistency and reducing inter-observer variability. The ATS became the subject of numerous validation studies, which confirmed its clinical robustness and its ability to predict major outcomes such as hospital admission, intensive care unit admission, and in-hospital mortality.

More than 30 years after its introduction, the Australasian Triage Scale remains one of the longest-standing and most consolidated triage models worldwide. Its evolution demonstrates the ability to adapt to epidemiological and organizational changes while maintaining a balance between methodological rigor, clinical practicality, and operational sustainability. The ATS is not only the matrix from which many other five-level systems have been derived but also a successful example of integration between scientific evidence and clinical practice, able to combine system efficiency with the centrality of nursing assessment [5, 8].

4.1.3 Objectives of the System

The ATS was conceived with a dual purpose. First, to ensure timely clinical assessment and accurate determination of patient severity [5, 7]. Second, to provide the emergency system with a tool for governance and monitoring of operational efficiency. From its introduction, the ATS has aimed to guarantee that no patient with a time-critical condition experiences delays in access to care, affirming the principle that the order of treatment must be determined by clinical urgency rather than arrival time [5, 7, 8].

The scale provides target assessment times for each urgency level, defining clear and measurable standards for clinical response [5, 8]. These time intervals do not have regulatory value but function as operational benchmarks to monitor how well services adhere to clinical priorities and to identify organizational weaknesses. The scale is also designed as a system interface linking nursing assessment to the overall functioning of the Emergency Department and triggering specific care pathways [8]. Each triage category thus becomes a measurement point for the quality of patient flow, allowing analysis of waiting times, workload, admission rates, and periodic review of performance using objective indicators.

The ATS also seeks to ensure inter-hospital consistency in urgency assessment. The presence of standardized criteria and clinical descriptors for each level reduces subjectivity, enabling greater uniformity of judgment among professionals and across organizational settings. To this end, the ATS is supported by dedicated educational programs designed to maintain consistent application over time and reduce inter-observer variability [5, 8].

Another key objective of the ATS is the dynamic nature of triage. The system recognizes that a patient's condition may change rapidly and considers regular reassessment an integral part of the process. This dynamic component allows priority to be updated according to clinical evolution, reducing the risk of initial under-triage and strengthening overall safety [5, 8]. Finally, the ATS introduces a perspective of professional accountability for the triage nurse, who is not a mere executor of protocols but a professional exercising clinical judgment supported by shared, validated criteria.

4.1.4　Clinical Functioning of the System

4.1.4.1 Operational Principles

The ATS is a five-category priority system. Each category corresponds to a target treatment time, defining the maximum interval within which the patient should be assessed by a physician and started on appropriate care. The system is simple yet rigorous, based on immediate clinical observation and nursing judgment supported by standardized criteria that guide rapid and as uniform as possible decision-making [5].

In practical terms, triage according to ATS is a professional clinical act based on observation and experience, centered on the nurse's reasoning [7, 10]. The triage nurse is required to integrate objective data, such as vital signs, level of consciousness, respiratory pattern, pain intensity, and mechanism of injury, with subjective and contextual clinical cues, such as general appearance, behavior, voice, and posture. Assessment must be rapid but structured, usually completed within 2–5 minutes, and its primary objective is to ensure that patients with time-critical conditions receive immediate attention [5, 8, 10].

The ATS is not an algorithm-driven system but a flexible decision-making framework that values clinical judgement and always recommends assigning the highest category compatible with the presentation [5, 7–10]. The guiding principle is clear: in case of doubt, choose the higher priority. The ATS also explicitly recognizes the dynamic nature of triage. Because clinical conditions may evolve quickly, the triage nurse has a duty to reassess patients in the waiting area periodically, upgrading the category if new signs of instability or deterioration emerge. This feature is one of the defining elements of the system and provides additional safety, particularly in crowded or high-pressure environments.

4.1.5   Acuity Levels

The five ATS categories are each associated with a treatment time window and a corresponding level of clinical urgency [5].

Category 1—Immediate: Patients in cardiorespiratory arrest or with immediate threat to life or vital organs who require immediate treatment and continuous monitoring, with simultaneous assessment and intervention.

Category 2—Emergency: Patients who are potentially unstable, whose condition may rapidly deteriorate, and who require treatment within 10 minutes. This category represents a critical boundary where timely intervention can significantly modify prognosis.

Category 3—Urgent: Patients who are currently stable but at risk of deterioration or with significant pain, requiring evaluation within 30 minutes. Although not immediately unstable, these patients require timely medical attention to prevent complications.

Category 4—Semi-Urgent: Patients with minor injuries or chronic conditions without signs of instability, to be assessed within 60 minutes. These patients can safely wait for an hour without significant risk of deterioration.

Category 5—Nonurgent: Patients with minor problems or non-acute chronic conditions who can wait up to 120 minutes without clinical risk. Examples include repeat prescriptions, medical certificates, minor dressings, or suture removal. Although representing the lowest priority, these patients are still monitored to ensure that no one is lost within the system.

This classification is graded rather than rigid, and the final priority is always determined by the actual condition of the patient, not by a presumed diagnosis. ACEM guidelines recommend considering the higher level whenever aggravating factors are present, such as severe pain, vital sign abnormalities, extreme age, comorbidities, or communication difficulties [5, 8].

4.1.6 Decision-Making Process: How the Acuity Level Is Assigned

Assignment of the triage category follows a logical but concise sequence of assessment stages that guide the triage nurse towards the appropriate priority code [5, 8, 11].

The first stage is the immediate assessment, the so-called "look test." At first contact, the nurse observes the patient, assessing posture, breathing, color, level of consciousness, and behavior. In the presence of signs of vital compromise, the patient is immediately assigned to Category 1 or 2. This assessment takes only a few seconds but is crucial for identifying manifest emergencies that cannot tolerate delay.

Once this initial phase is completed, the presenting problem is collected. The triage nurse identifies the main reason that led the patient to seek care, for example, chest pain, dyspnea, trauma, or fever, and evaluates its clinical relevance in light of the overall presentation, formulating an initial professional impression. Although the ATS does not include a codified list or strictly structured symptom-based pathways, recognition of the presenting problem provides a clinical frame of reference, linking the reported symptom to possible severity and enabling an early estimation of the most appropriate urgency level. In practice, the symptom and its severity, interpreted by the nurse in the context of clinical observation, form the basis upon which objective vital-sign assessment, general appearance, and perceived risk of rapid deterioration are integrated [5, 8].

The nurse then proceeds to evaluate vital signs and key symptoms. After identifying the presenting problem, a multiparametric assessment is performed, measuring heart rate, respiratory rate, blood pressure, oxygen saturation, and mental status. These objective data are interpreted within the clinical context defined by the main symptom, which provides the alarm framework and guides the reading of values. In other words, vital signs are not considered in isolation but weighed in relation to the overall presentation. Significant abnormalities, such as marked tachycardia, hypotension, tachypnea, or reduced level of consciousness, are indicators of instability and automatically lead to assignment of a higher priority level. The goal is not merely to record numbers but to capture their clinical meaning in relation to the observed picture, confirming or correcting the initial impression provided by the presenting symptom [5, 8, 11].

In parallel with vital-sign assessment, pain evaluation is performed. Pain is considered a clinically and humanly relevant parameter. Its intensity, measured using numerical or analog scales, can raise the priority even in the absence of vital sign instability. A patient with severe pain, rated above seven out of ten, may be placed in a higher category than that suggested by the clinical presentation alone, recognizing that intense pain is itself an emergency requiring prompt treatment.

Integration of all these elements leads to category assignment. The ATS category represents the final synthesis of the triage nurse's clinical reasoning. After integrating the presenting problem, general observation, and objective data, the nurse assigns the priority level that reflects the most serious condition identified. The aim is not to strike a compromise among indicators but to recognize the most urgent clinical manifestation and use it as the decision reference. The assigned category must therefore represent the highest plausible risk, ensuring that no potentially unstable patient is underestimated. In the presence of doubts or discrepancies between vital signs and clinical impression, the decision must always be conservative and safety-oriented. Once assigned, the category is recorded together with its clinical rationale, marking the start of the target time for medical assessment [5, 8].

The final stage of the process is reassessment and documentation. The ATS requires ongoing monitoring of the patient after category assignment to anticipate possible changes in condition. Monitoring of the target time is initiated, and periodic reassessments are scheduled until the patient is seen. This apparently linear process is underpinned by complex professional competence, requiring experience, clinical sensitivity, and deep knowledge of vital-sign behavior across age groups and pathological conditions.

4.1.6.1 Development and Internal Validation

From the outset, development of the ATS was accompanied by an internal verification process to ensure that the system, in addition to being conceptually sound, functioned effectively in the real-world practice of Australian emergency departments [5, 8]. The ACEM working group did not merely propose a tabletop theoretical scale; rather, it undertook multicenter field testing to verify coherence, reproducibility, and discriminative ability [5, 8, 10, 11].

The five priority levels and their associated target times, from immediate to 120 minutes, were not chosen arbitrarily but emerged from empirical analysis of real ED data. ACEM collected actual treatment times and clinical outcomes from thousands of attendances, observing that conditions with critical outcomes, such as cardiac arrest, shock, and severe respiratory failure, required immediate or near-immediate intervention, whereas intermediate urgencies could safely wait up to 30 minutes without compromising prognosis [5, 8, 10, 11]. These observations led to the definition of five progressive temporal thresholds corresponding to increasing gradients of risk and urgency.

In parallel, the working group collected and analyzed the most frequent clinical presentations in EDs and compared them with observed outcomes such as hospital admission, intensive care, life-saving interventions, and early mortality. From this mapping exercise emerged the exemplar clinical descriptors for the five categories, still reported in official documents and subsequently updated over time [5, 8, 10, 11]. Associations between symptom and priority were derived from clinical observation and validated through professional consensus rather than formal statistical modeling.

After preliminary construction, the ATS was piloted in several centers to verify internal coherence and reproducibility. The initial applications aimed to determine whether the defined levels corresponded to the actual degree of clinical urgency and whether they could be applied uniformly by different operators. Analysis of collected cases demonstrated a direct relationship between assigned level and clinical complexity, confirming that the higher categories identified patients with greater likelihood of hospitalization, life-saving interventions, and critical outcomes.

In summary, the development and internal validation of the ATS were based on an empirical and participatory approach in which clinical experience, observation of real-world data, and professional consensus produced a coherent, reproducible, and easy-to-use system [5, 8, 10, 11]. The association between priority levels and target times was supported by clinical outcomes, while the definition of category descriptors allowed standardization of professional judgment without eliminating its interpretive component. The success of this testing phase enabled ACEM to approve the nationwide implementation of the ATS as the national standard, marking the birth of the first triage system officially validated and shared across the Australasian region.

4.1.7   External Validation After Implementation

Following its official adoption as a national standard, the ATS underwent numerous external validation processes aimed at evaluating its reliability, consistency of application, and ability to correctly discriminate clinical severity. These assessments, conducted both in Australia and internationally, were crucial in consolidating its scientific value and defining the system's operational limits.

Inter-observer reliability, that is, the degree to which different operators assign the same category to the same case, has generally been found to be moderate, with kappa values around 0.428 [10]. This variability is closely linked to the core structure of the system, which assigns a major role to the triage nurse and is therefore influenced by differences in operational context and staff training [10–12]. Studies based on large samples of simulated or real cases have confirmed that consistency increases substantially among experienced operators or after dedicated training programs. Concordance is highest at the extremes, Categories 1 and 5, where severity or normality is most evident, whereas disagreement is more frequent in intermediate categories (2–4), where clinical judgement and subjective risk interpretation play a greater role [7, 10]. These findings have reinforced the understanding that triage nurse competence is an integral component of system validity and that ongoing education is essential to maintain reliability.

In terms of validity, defined as the system's ability to predict tangible outcomes, the ATS has demonstrated a strong relationship between assigned category and real clinical outcomes, confirming its capacity to discriminate patient severity [1, 2, 13, 14]. Patients classified in Categories 1 and 2 exhibit significantly higher rates of ED mortality and life-saving interventions compared with lower categories, whereas Categories 4 and 5 are associated in most cases with direct discharge and lower resource consumption [1, 2]. This progressive pattern has been observed in multiple independent studies, confirming that the scale effectively reproduces the expected relationship between clinical urgency and care intensity.

Nonetheless, some areas of concern have been identified. Conditions with subtle initial presentations may occasionally be underestimated, particularly when vital signs at presentation remain stable. These cases constitute examples of physiological under-triage linked to the intrinsic limits of an assessment based on observable status at first contact rather than explicit interrogation of the underlying pathophysiology [1, 2, 14]. Revisions by ACEM have therefore emphasized the need for dynamic reassessment and heightened attention to weak or evolving signals, reinforcing the view of triage as a continuous process [15].

Post-implementation evaluations have also confirmed that the ATS maintains good adherence to target treatment times, albeit with variability related to workload and resource availability [1, 2, 9, 12–14]. The concept of "fractile performance," introduced in early guidelines, has proved a useful tool for monitoring triage quality, enabling assessment not only of individual compliance with time targets but also of the system's overall capacity to provide access proportionate to clinical need. Overall, external validations have confirmed the clinical robustness and operational reliability of the Australasian Triage Scale, demonstrating that it orders patients in a manner consistent with actual severity and produces a priority gradient that translates into progressive and measurable clinical outcomes [13].

4.1.8   Role of the Triage Nurse

Within the ATS framework, the triage nurse occupies an absolutely central position [5, 7, 11]. The system was conceived from the outset as clinician-led, with explicit recognition of nursing expertise. The triage nurse does not merely execute an algorithm; rather, triage is an autonomous act of clinical judgement, regulated by shared criteria but applied through contextual and individualized assessment. The ATS acknowledges that patient presentation cannot be interpreted univocally and that priority depends on multiple factors, symptoms, physiological stability, risk of deterioration, and required resources that must be rapidly and competently synthesized by the triage nurse [5, 7, 11].

In the absence of an automatic correspondence between symptom and level, the system relies on the nurse's ability to interpret the presenting problem, evaluate vital signs and assign the most appropriate ATS category based on perceived severity and potential clinical evolution. This approach grants the triage nurse considerable decisional latitude but also a high level of professional responsibility. ACEM recommendations emphasize key elements: advanced clinical competence derived from substantial frontline experience, specific training in ATS, ability to integrate objective data with perceived risk, and awareness of the direct impact that triage decisions have on patient safety and flow efficiency [5, 16].

This configuration differentiates the triage nurse's role under ATS from that in other models such as MTS or ESI. Whereas those systems are partly guided by algorithms, the ATS relies primarily on the triage nurse's competence as the main risk-discrimination tool. It is the nurse who, through experience and clinical sensitivity, determines urgency, deciding whether a borderline condition warrants an upgrade in priority for safety reasons. Subjectivity of judgment is not viewed as a limitation but as an intrinsic component of nursing professionalism. However, to contain variability, ACEM has consistently highlighted the importance of continuous education, audit sessions, and interprofessional discussion as essential tools for maintaining uniform application and ensuring that discretion translates into precision rather than arbitrariness [16].

In summary, within the ATS the triage nurse is both clinical decision-maker and safety guarantor: they interpret the patient's condition, apply priority criteria, and directly influence the quality of the care pathway. Through their assessment, the system preserves its flexibility, adapting to the infinite variability of emergency practice without losing coherence or reliability.

4.1.9 Special Populations

The ATS recognizes that uniform application of priority criteria may be inadequate for certain clinical populations whose physiology, symptom presentation, or ability to communicate distress differs from typical adult patterns [5, 16, 17]. While the decision-making structure of the system remains unchanged, the ATS introduces specific recommendations for pediatric patients and pregnant women [5, 17].

Pediatrics is one of the main areas of focus. From its earliest guidelines, the ATS acknowledged that pediatric vital signs differ markedly from adult values and that children's ability to express pain or discomfort may be limited [5]. Dedicated pediatric descriptors have therefore been developed, maintaining the five priority categories but with age-adjusted physiological ranges and clinical signs. The role of a dedicated pediatric triage nurse is also envisaged, emphasizing observation of general appearance, such as activity level, color and interaction, respiratory behavior, response to pain, and parental input. The aim is to reduce the risk of underestimating severity, particularly in infants and nonverbal children, in whom deterioration can be rapid and subtle. Although not configured as a separate system, as with the Canadian Paediatric CTAS, the pediatric ATS represents an integrated and adapted version that remains coherent with the original structure while being sensitive to the physiological and communicative specificities of developmental age.

For pregnant women, the ATS recommends that each patient be assessed with explicit consideration of the cardiovascular, respiratory, and metabolic adaptations of pregnancy, which can alter the interpretation of vital signs and mask compromise [17]. Guidelines emphasize that the presence of abdominal pain, vaginal bleeding, or altered consciousness during pregnancy should lead to immediate escalation of priority, even in the absence of frankly abnormal vital signs. The triage nurse must therefore consider pregnancy as a risk-amplifying factor, adopting a precautionary approach and ensuring that assessment includes, when necessary, prompt consultation with an obstetrician or an emergency physician with obstetric expertise.

4.1.10 Strengths and Clinical Advantages

The ATS has maintained its position as a reference among international triage systems due to a combination of simplicity, reliability, and adaptability. Its linear architecture, grounded in empirical data and continuously updated through professional discussion, constitutes the core of the model. The ATS has proven able to provide rapid, consistent, and clinically justifiable prioritization, with good reproducibility even in high-pressure environments.

One of its main advantages is operational immediacy. The ATS was designed to be used in real time without the need for complex algorithms or specific electronic tools. This enables the triage nurse to make quick decisions based on clinical observation, vital signs, and expert judgment. The resulting speed, combined with clear descriptors, reduces assessment time and optimizes patient flow, particularly in high-throughput or resource-limited settings. The simplicity of the system does not compromise clinical accuracy; rather, it reduces the risk of errors linked to complicated procedures or lack of specialized tools.

The balance between standardization and clinical flexibility is another defining characteristic. Alongside clear, shared reference criteria, the system allows room for professional judgment, recognizing that risk assessment cannot be fully codified. This approach makes it possible to adapt triage to a wide range of scenarios—from major trauma to general medical conditions—while maintaining methodological consistency without introducing operational rigidity. At the same time, it enables management of borderline cases in which the operator's sensitivity and experience can be decisive for appropriate diagnostic orientation and prioritization.

From an organizational perspective, the ATS stands out for its integration with performance-monitoring mechanisms. The target times associated with each level constitute measurable quality indicators that allow evaluation of the ED's ability to respond equitably and promptly to clinical needs. Thus, the scale functions not only as a clinical tool but also as a governance device, useful for analyzing service efficiency, identifying flow bottlenecks, and planning improvement interventions. The concept of fractile performance, measuring the proportion of patients seen within target times, provides a robust and clinically meaningful indicator of system quality [5, 16].

Another advantage lies in structured and standardized training. ACEM has consistently supported uniform educational programs, guidelines, and training materials that have ensured high coherence of application nationally [16, 18]. This investment in professional competence has strengthened the role of the triage nurse as clinical decision-maker and has helped evolve triage from an administrative act into an advanced assessment process. The availability of structured educational materials, standardized clinical cases, and certification programs has made it possible to maintain high competence standards even in settings with staff turnover.

In summary, the strengths of the ATS reside in its methodological simplicity, empirical foundation, and emphasis on clinical judgment, features that have underpinned its longevity and operational effectiveness. It is a system that has successfully combined the scientific rigor of prioritization with the practical realities of emergency care, providing a balanced, realistic, and sustainable model for modern emergency-urgency management.

4.1.11 Limitations and Clinical Disadvantages

The ATS also has limitations that partially affect its discriminative precision and its transferability to contexts different from the Australasian setting. The system's main strength, the central role of nurse clinical judgment, also represents its principal vulnerability. The ATS relies heavily on the autonomy of the triage nurse, who integrates clinical observation, vital signs, and perceived risk to assign priority. This approach confers great flexibility and adaptive capacity but exposes the system to a high degree of subjectivity [10].

Unlike more structured models such as ESI or MTS, which are based on stepwise decision algorithms, the ATS depends strongly on the individual operator's experience and intuition. While this feature valorizes professionalism, it may lead to inter-observer variability and reduced reproducibility of acuity levels, particularly in borderline cases. Validation studies have indeed shown that the ATS has slightly lower discriminative ability than other systems, with overall good but somewhat inferior sensitivity and specificity compared with more analytical models like ESI and MTS [1, 2, 19]. A plausible explanation is the absence of strict decision constraints and the predominance of individual judgment over objective data. In other words, the interpretive freedom at the heart of the model can, under certain conditions, become a source of methodological fragility.

A second limitation is the lack of built-in decision support tools such as integrated risk scores or predefined symptom pathways. The ATS provides exemplar clinical descriptors but does not offer structured algorithms for specific presenting complaints, leaving the triage nurse responsible for interpreting and weighing each case. While this ensures flexibility, it increases the risk of under-triage in atypical presentations and may generate behavioral differences between centers with varying levels of experience or resources. The absence of explicit decision pathways for specific clinical presentations makes the system less suitable for settings with less experienced staff or marked variability in training.

From an operational standpoint, maintaining consistent application in high-load environments is another challenge. In situations of overcrowding or staff shortages, the rapid judgment required by the system can accentuate variability and reduce consistency among triage nurses. In addition, it is difficult to monitor decision quality precisely, as the ATS audit framework, based on compliance with target times via fractile performance, measures organizational efficiency but does not always capture the clinical correctness of assigned priorities. This may result in scenarios where time targets are met but the quality of classification is suboptimal.

Finally, the ATS has limitations in terms of transparency of decision criteria. Because the system relies heavily on expert judgement, it can sometimes be difficult to retrospectively explain why a specific level was assigned, particularly when the clinical presentation changes rapidly. This can complicate error analysis and hinder continuous improvement of triage processes. The lack of explicit traceability of clinical reasoning may also create challenges in audit or medico-legal review, where justification of decisions is critical for professional protection and organizational learning.

4.2 South African Triage Scale (SATS)

4.2.1 Introduction

The South African Triage Scale (SATS) represents one of the most innovative and pragmatic responses to the challenges of triage in settings characterized by high patient volumes, limited resources, and staff with heterogeneous levels of experience [20]. Born from the concrete need to manage the pressure on South African emergency departments, SATS stands out for its hybrid architecture, which combines parametric objectivity with clinical flexibility, offering a tool that is at once simple to apply and clinically reliable [20].

The underlying philosophy of SATS rests on a fundamental principle: to provide a standardized and reproducible instrument that enables patients to be ordered according to their actual clinical urgency, ensuring timely care even when the demand for services significantly exceeds the system's response capacity [20, 21]. This feature has made SATS particularly suitable not only for its original South African context but also for international scenarios in which the imbalance between healthcare needs and available resources is a daily challenge [20, 21].

SATS is characterized by a deliberately linear and sequential decision-making approach, which minimizes interpretative subjectivity while preserving room for expert clinical judgment. Its structure is built around two main components: the physiological score TEWS (Triage Early Warning Score) and clinical discriminators [20]. Together, these allow the system to capture both manifest physiological instability and high-risk conditions that may not be immediately evident from vital signs alone [20].

A distinctive element of SATS is its operational vocation: it does not simply classify patients but directly guides the allocation of space and resources through a streaming system that links priority levels to the functional areas of the ED (resuscitation, high-acuity area, minor area) [20, 21]. This integration between clinical assessment and flow management makes it a particularly effective tool in daily practice.

The diffusion of SATS beyond South Africa's borders testifies to its versatility and adaptability [22]. The system has been implemented in several African countries, in both hospital and prehospital settings, and has proved especially useful in humanitarian and mass-casualty emergencies, where rapid decision-making and operational simplicity are essential for effective patient flow management [20, 22, 23].

4.2.2 History: Origin, Context of Development and Evolution

SATS emerged in the mid-2000s within a South African health system facing unique and complex challenges. Post-apartheid South Africa was navigating a difficult transition, with huge disparities in access to care, an uneven distribution of resources between urban and rural areas, and a population with a distinctive epidemiological profile, marked by the coexistence of diseases typical of high-income countries (cardiovascular disease, cancer) and those of low- and middle-income settings (infectious diseases, malnutrition, and trauma) [20, 23].

The working group that developed SATS consisted mainly of emergency physicians and nurses working daily in these high-pressure environments [20]. Their direct frontline experience was decisive in shaping the system's characteristics: it had to be rapid to apply, based on objective and easily reproducible criteria, usable by staff with varying levels of training, and robust enough to remain reliable even under conditions of crowding.

The influence of existing international triage systems is evident in SATS' structure, but its originality lies in the intelligent adaptation to specific operational constraints. While systems such as CTAS and ATS required highly specialized nurses and relatively long assessment times, SATS was designed to be applicable even by staff with less specialist training, while still maintaining high safety standards.

The first implementation of SATS took place in pilot hospitals in the Western Cape region, where preliminary results showed a significant reduction in waiting times for high-priority patients and improved resource utilization. These encouraging findings led to a gradual expansion of the system to other South African provinces.

The evolution of SATS has been characterized by a pragmatic, evidence-oriented approach. The initial version was continuously refined based on clinical experience and internal audit results. In 2006, the first standardized version was published, followed by the pediatric version (PaedSATS), developed in collaboration with pediatric emergency specialists [20, 24, 25].

A crucial milestone in SATS' evolution was its adoption by the South African Department of Health as the national standard for hospital triage. This official recognition led to the development of structured training programs, detailed operational manuals, and quality-monitoring systems.

International expansion began around 2010, when humanitarian organizations started using SATS in emergency settings [22]. Its operational simplicity and ability to function effectively with limited resources made it particularly attractive for crisis interventions. Countries such as Kenya and Tanzania subsequently adopted adapted versions of SATS as part of their national health systems [26, 27].

The international scientific community has recognized the value of SATS through numerous publications validating its effectiveness in diverse contexts [20, 26, 27]. This body of evidence has contributed to its dissemination and stimulated further research to optimize its use in specific scenarios.

4.2.3 System Objectives

SATS was conceived with clear, measurable objectives that reflect the specific challenges of the environments in which it is meant to operate [20].

The primary objective is the early identification of patients who cannot safely wait, ensuring that time-critical conditions receive absolute priority regardless of arrival volume or momentary organizational pressure [20, 28]. The combination of clinical discriminators and a physiological score is specifically calibrated to maximize sensitivity for these critical conditions.

A second key objective is to maintain effectiveness under conditions of extreme organizational stress. Unlike other triage systems whose reliability may deteriorate as workload increases, SATS was designed to remain functional during demand surges, crowding, or staff shortages [26, 29]. This operational resilience is achieved through simple decision criteria and a rapid assessment process.

Another fundamental aim is to reduce inter-operator variability in priority assignment [30]. Before SATS, patient classification depended largely on the individual experience and subjective judgement of the operator, leading to significant inconsistencies that could jeopardize safety [20, 30]. SATS seeks to standardize decision-making through explicit criteria and objective parameters, minimizing arbitrary interpretation.

4.2.4 Clinical Functioning of the System

SATS is distinguished by an intentionally linear, structured decision-making process designed to minimize operational complexity while preserving high clinical accuracy [20, 31]. Its architecture is based on a logical sequence of assessments that proceeds in successive steps, each of which can directly determine the final priority level or direct the process to the next step [20, 31].

The process always starts with an immediate evaluation to identify obvious signs of life-threatening emergency, which mandate direct transfer to the resuscitation area with no further triage steps [20, 31]. This initial "first look" phase is crucial for promptly recognizing conditions that require immediate intervention: cardiorespiratory arrest, overt shock, severe airway compromise, and major neurological derangement [20, 31].

In the absence of manifest life-threatening emergencies, the system proceeds with the application of clinical discriminators, key elements representing specific signs, symptoms, or conditions that automatically confer a high priority, regardless of current vital signs [20, 31]. These discriminators were selected based on their ability to identify high-risk or time-dependent conditions.

When no clinical discriminators apply, the parametric component of the system is activated via the Triage Early Warning Score (TEWS) [20, 32]. This score integrates major vital signs and indicators of physiological stability, generating a quantitative estimate of the patient's status that directly translates into a priority category.

The system also provides for clinician-initiated, justified overrides, recognizing that complex clinical scenarios may not be fully captured by standardized criteria. This controlled flexibility preserves clinical judgment as an essential component of the decision process.

4.2.5 Acuity Levels

SATS uses a five-level color-coded classification, each level associated with specific time targets that define the urgency of medical evaluation. This color structure facilitates immediate communication and shared understanding of priorities among all healthcare staff [20, 21].

RED (Emergency): Highest priority, requiring immediate treatment. Patients present an imminent threat to life or to vital functions and cannot tolerate any delay.

ORANGE (Very Urgent): Patients who must be evaluated within 10 minutes of arrival. This group includes serious or potentially unstable conditions that, while not requiring instantaneous intervention, cannot safely wait without a significant risk of deterioration.

YELLOW (Urgent): Target assessment time of 60 minutes. Includes patients who require timely medical evaluation but can wait without immediate risk of worsening.

GREEN (Less Urgent): Assessment within 4 hours. Patients with minor conditions or exacerbations of chronic disease without short-term risk of deterioration.

BLUE (Dead): Administrative category for patients who are deceased on arrival or who die while in the Emergency Department. It requires administrative management within 2 hours for medico-legal and organizational reasons. It is not a clinical priority category but a specific management requirement.

These time frames are not rigid maximum limits but operational targets used to evaluate system performance and identify organizational bottlenecks.

4.2.6 How the Acuity Level Is Assigned

The priority-assignment process in SATS follows a structured decision sequence that combines immediate clinical observation, application of specific discriminators, and quantitative parametric assessment [20, 21].

I. Immediate Emergency Assessment

The process begins with a rapid visual assessment at arrival. This phase, which should last only a few seconds, aims to identify obvious signs of vital compromise requiring immediate intervention. Findings such as cyanosis, agonal breathing, loss of consciousness, massive hemorrhage, or abnormal posturing lead to immediate assignment of RED and direct transfer to the resuscitation area.

II. Application of Clinical Discriminators

In the absence of evident life-threatening emergencies, the triage nurse checks for specific clinical discriminators, signs, symptoms, or conditions that, due to their nature or associated risk of deterioration, automatically entail a high priority (RED, ORANGE, or YELLOW). These discriminators are grouped by category, for example: cardiovascular, respiratory, neurological, trauma, and infectious.

The presence of any discriminator leads to the assignment of ORANGE or a higher priority, regardless of current vital signs.

III. Calculation of TEWS

When no clinical discriminators are present, vital signs are measured and the TEWS is calculated. The score typically includes: Respiratory rate, systolic blood pressure, heart rate, body temperature, level of consciousness (AVPU), mobility, and presence and severity of trauma.

Each parameter is assigned points according to its deviation from normal ranges. The total TEWS determines the priority: 0–1 points equal GREEN; 2–4 points equal YELLOW; 5–6 points equal ORANGE; $\geq$7 points equal RED [20, 21].

IV. Integration and Clinical Override

The final priority level is determined by the most urgent result between clinical discriminators and TEWS. The system explicitly allows justified clinical override when the experienced professional judges that the standard criteria do not adequately reflect the patient's risk.

V. Reassessment

In SATS, triage is conceived as a dynamic process. Waiting patients must be reassessed periodically, at intervals determined by the initial priority: ORANGE every 15 minutes, YELLOW every 30 minutes, and GREEN every hour. Reassessment may lead to upgrading or downgrading the priority according to the clinical evolution.

4.2.7 Development and Internal Validation

SATS is a paradigmatic example of a triage system developed through a pragmatic, practice-oriented approach without sacrificing methodological rigor [20]. From the outset, its construction was guided by the need for a tool that would work effectively under real-world conditions in South African emergency departments, high volumes, limited resources, and staff with heterogeneous training [20, 21].

The multidisciplinary working group adopted a methodology based on available evidence and direct clinical experience. The initial phase consisted of an in-depth analysis of existing international triage systems, particularly their performance in settings similar to South Africa. This review showed that many systems, although clinically valid, had major limitations when applied in high-pressure, resource-constrained environments.

The decision to use a hybrid approach combining clinical discriminators and a physiological score arose from the observation that neither strategy alone could fully capture the complexity of emergency presentations. Clinical discriminators were excellent at identifying specific high-risk conditions but could miss critical cases with atypical presentations. Physiological scores were sensitive to general instability but could underestimate time-critical conditions with initially normal vital signs.

The clinical discriminators were defined on the basis of a retrospective analysis of thousands of cases from several South African hospitals. Presentations showing the strongest association with adverse outcomes (mortality, life-saving intervention, ICU admission, rapid clinical deterioration) were identified. This analysis allowed the selection of a set of discriminators that maximized sensitivity for critical conditions while maintaining acceptable specificity.

The development of TEWS represented a major innovation [20, 32]. Building on the concept of Early Warning Scores used in inpatient wards, the group adapted the tool to the triage context, modifying the included parameters, normal ranges, and scoring system. Internal validation of TEWS was carried out through a prospective study, demonstrating a strong correlation between TEWS and relevant clinical outcomes.

A distinctive aspect of SATS construction was the emphasis on operational feasibility. Every component of the system was tested under real working conditions, assessing not only clinical accuracy but also ease of use, application time, and reproducibility among operators with varying levels of experience [20, 33]. This operational testing led to multiple refinements, streamlining complex procedures and removing elements that proved impractical in daily use [20, 21, 33].

Internal validation included structured research programs: inter-observer agreement studies, which showed weighted kappa coefficients above 0.75 for all priority levels; predictive validity studies, which confirmed that SATS effectively stratifies patients by risk and correlates with outcomes such as admission, ICU transfer, and mortality [20, 21, 30].

4.2.8   External Validation

Following its initial implementation in South Africa, SATS underwent extensive external validation to test its effectiveness, reliability, and transferability across diverse geographic and operational settings [24, 26–28]. This process was crucial for establishing the system's scientific credibility and for identifying optimal implementation conditions.

The first external validation studies were conducted in other African countries with health systems similar to South Africa's. A multicenter study in Ghana, Kenya, and Tanzania, showed that SATS maintained its performance characteristics in different cultural and organizational contexts [24, 25, 27, 28].

The pediatric component (PaedSATS) was validated in specific studies [25]. Multicenter validation studies showed sensitivity >90% for critical conditions and negative predictive value of about 95% for predicting admission [25].

The scientific literature has also highlighted some limitations, such as lower sensitivity for certain conditions compared with more complex systems. Nonetheless, these limitations were generally considered acceptable in light of the system's operational advantages and the possibility of mitigation through targeted training.

4.2.9   Role of the Triage Nurse

Within SATS, the triage nurse occupies a central, multidimensional role that goes well beyond the mechanical application of standardized criteria. The philosophy of SATS recognizes the nurse as a competent clinical professional capable of integrating objective assessment with professional judgment to ensure safety and efficiency in triage [20, 34].

Technical competencies include full mastery of the decision pathway, from immediate emergency assessment to the application of more complex clinical discriminators [20, 34]. The nurse must accurately measure vital signs, calculate TEWS rapidly, and correctly interpret results in the clinical context. The ability to recognize early warning signs of deterioration and apply override criteria appropriately is particularly important [20, 34].

A distinctive aspect of the nursing role in SATS is responsibility for dynamic reassessment. Unlike more static systems, SATS requires the triage nurse to maintain active surveillance over waiting patients, periodically reassessing their condition and changing priority when necessary. This demands strong organizational skills and the ability to manage multiple patients simultaneously without losing sight of key clinical details [20].

Communication is another essential competency. The triage nurse must clearly explain the triage process, expected waiting times, and reasons for assigned priorities to patients and families. In high-volume settings, good communication can significantly reduce tension and conflict.

The nurse also bears specific documentation responsibilities: recording all assessment elements (vital signs, applied discriminators, TEWS, and assigned priority), documenting reassessments and overrides, and tracking times to enable performance monitoring. Documentation is not merely administrative but an essential tool for clinical audit and continuous quality improvement.

SATS further expects experienced triage nurses to play an educational and mentoring role for less experienced colleagues, especially during system roll-out or when staff turnover is high.

Finally, the emotional and cognitive load of the role is explicitly recognized. Triage nurses under SATS often work under intense pressure, must make rapid decisions with potentially major consequences, and must handle the anxiety and expectations of patients and families. The system therefore encourages support measures such as debriefing and psychological support. Continuous education, through updates, case-based training, and participation in clinical audits, is considered essential to maintain high levels of competence in a constantly evolving clinical landscape [26, 34–36].

4.2.10 Special Populations

SATS demonstrates its versatility and completeness through the attention devoted to special populations, acknowledging that certain patient groups require tailored assessment approaches while maintaining alignment with the general decision structure. This adaptability is one of SATS' strengths and supports its use in diverse clinical contexts.

The pediatric version, PaedSATS, is a sophisticated adaptation developed in collaboration with pediatric emergency specialists and validated in studies involving thousands of children [25]. PaedSATS preserves the core decision architecture of the adult system but introduces substantial modifications reflecting the physiological and clinical peculiarities of pediatric patients.

Vital signs in PaedSATS are stratified into age-specific bands, recognizing that normal values for heart rate, respiratory rate, and blood pressure vary considerably from birth to adolescence [25]. Pediatric clinical discriminators include specific elements such as inconsolable irritability, reduced social responsiveness, altered feeding patterns, and specific signs of dehydration. Particular emphasis is placed on early signs of pediatric sepsis, given its central role in child mortality where SATS is most often applied.

PaedSATS also incorporates behavioral observation scales to objectively assess the child's level of compromise by observing interaction with caregivers, response to stimuli, and overall activity level, especially useful in young children who cannot communicate verbally.

Management of pregnant patients under SATS follows specific principles that consider both maternal and fetal well-being [20]. The system includes obstetric discriminators for conditions such as antepartum hemorrhage, pre-eclampsia/eclampsia, preterm labor, premature rupture of membranes, and reduced fetal movements [20, 37].

Vital signs in pregnancy are interpreted in light of physiological changes for each trimester, with particular attention to blood pressure because gestational hypertension can rapidly evolve into severe complications.

4.2.11 Strengths and Clinical Advantages

SATS offers numerous strengths that distinguish it among international triage systems and make it particularly suitable for complex, heterogeneous operational contexts [20]. These advantages derive from its hybrid architecture, operational simplicity, and pragmatic design philosophy.

One of the main strengths is the balance between standardization and clinical judgment [20]. By effectively combining objective criteria (TEWS) with specific clinical discriminators, SATS creates a framework that reduces inter-operator variability while preserving space for professional expertise [20]. This is particularly valuable in environments where staff have diverse experience levels: less-experienced clinicians can rely on structured criteria, while experts retain the ability to exercise clinical judgment when appropriate.

The TEWS component provides a robust quantitative basis for assessment, eliminating much of the subjectivity that characterizes other triage systems. At the same time, clinical discriminators capture high-risk conditions that may not be immediately apparent from vital signs alone. Together, these components maximize both sensitivity for critical conditions and specificity for low-risk patients.

Another major advantage is the system's operational simplicity and low technological demand. SATS was designed from the outset to function effectively in resource-limited environments. It does not require sophisticated equipment, advanced IT systems, or highly specialized personnel. This makes it ideal for rural hospitals, peripheral health centers, humanitarian emergencies, and mass-casualty situations where technology may be limited or absent [26–28].

Simplicity does not come at the expense of clinical accuracy. On the contrary, reducing operational complexity decreases the risk of errors associated with cumbersome procedures or lack of specific tools.

Another clear strength is speed of application. The decision process is designed to be completed within a few minutes, an essential feature in high-volume settings where triage time must be minimized to avoid bottlenecks. The linear sequence of assessments often allows a decision to be reached even before all steps are completed, further accelerating the process.

4.2.12 Limitations and Clinical Disadvantages

Despite its many strengths, SATS also has limitations and critical aspects that must be recognized and managed to optimize its effectiveness. These do not necessarily undermine the system's overall utility but require awareness and mitigation strategies.

One of the main limitations concerns performance in conditions that present with subtle or atypical early symptoms [34, 38]. Early sepsis, pulmonary embolism, non-ST-elevation myocardial infarction, and some forms of stroke may initially show normal or only mildly altered vital signs and may not meet criteria for specific clinical discriminators.

Similarly, pulmonary embolism may present with mild dyspnea, atypical chest pain, and normal vital signs, particularly in young patients with good cardiopulmonary reserve. SATS may classify these patients as YELLOW or even GREEN, potentially delaying diagnosis and treatment of a life-threatening condition [38].

A second critical issue concerns the risk of over-triage. SATS tends to produce relatively high over-triage rates, especially when applied by less-experienced staff or in high-pressure environments [38]. While this may provide a safety buffer from a clinical perspective, it can have significant organizational consequences.

Over-triage leads to assigning higher priorities than necessary to patients with relatively benign conditions, overloading high-intensity care areas, and resulting in suboptimal resource use. In already strained settings, this may paradoxically increase waiting times for truly critical patients and reduce overall system efficiency.

This phenomenon is particularly evident in the application of clinical discriminators, where subjective interpretation can lead to over-liberal use of criteria. For example, the chest-pain discriminator may be applied to patients with clearly musculoskeletal pain, resulting in inappropriate ORANGE assignments.

For these reasons, careful training, ongoing supervision, and regular audits are essential components of SATS implementation in order to mitigate these limitations and maintain an appropriate balance between patient safety and operational efficiency [36].

4.3   Emergency Severity Index (ESI)

4.3.1   Introduction

The Emergency Severity Index (ESI) is one of the most significant innovations in the international landscape of triage systems, distinguished by a conceptual approach that goes beyond traditional classifications based solely on clinical urgency [1, 2, 39]. Developed in the late 1990s in the United States, the ESI introduced a completely new paradigm in hospital triage by combining the assessment of clinical acuity with the prediction of diagnostic and therapeutic resource use [39]. It thus provides a tool that simultaneously addresses both the clinical and operational needs of modern EDs.

The underlying philosophy of the ESI rests on a key principle: triage should not merely rank patients according to clinical severity but also support efficient resource allocation and the organization of care pathways [39, 40]. This integrated vision has made the ESI particularly suitable for the U.S. healthcare setting, characterized by very high-volume EDs, complex organizational structures, and strong economic pressure to optimize resource use [39–41].

The ESI architecture is notable for its operational simplicity. It is based on a linear decision algorithm that uses binary questions to guide the triage nurse through a structured yet rapid process [39–41]. This feature makes it especially attractive in settings where processing speed is crucial for flow management, without compromising the accuracy of clinical assessment.

A distinctive element of the ESI is its differentiated approach to time targets. Unlike other systems that specify time goals for all priority levels, the ESI focuses temporal targets on the most critical patients (levels 1 and 2), whereas for lower levels it prioritizes organization by resource intensity instead of strict time urgency [39–41]. This choice reflects a sophisticated understanding of ED dynamics, where efficient management of stable patients is just as important as rapid intervention for the critically ill [39–41].

The ESI has shown a remarkable capacity for adaptation and dissemination, being implemented not only in the United States but also in several other countries, often within predominantly private healthcare systems, where it has been adapted to local specificities [40, 41].

The scientific robustness of the ESI is supported by a large body of evidence that has validated its effectiveness in different operational contexts. Studies have confirmed its ability to predict not only traditional clinical outcomes but also key operational parameters such as resource consumption and care complexity, thereby confirming the validity of its integrated approach [39–41].

4.3.2   History: Origins, Context of Development, and Evolution

The ESI emerged in a particular historical phase for U.S. emergency medicine, marked by profound changes in the national healthcare landscape [39]. The 1990s saw an exponential increase in ED visits, driven by multiple factors: population ageing, the rise of complex chronic diseases, reduced access to primary care and, paradoxically, improvements in diagnostic and therapeutic capabilities in EDs, which made them increasingly attractive to patients [39].

The U.S. healthcare context of that period was also characterized by growing economic pressure. The introduction of Diagnosis Related Groups (DRGs) and the spread of managed care organizations created an environment in which operational efficiency and optimal resource management became crucial for the financial sustainability of hospitals. EDs were therefore required to balance the clinical imperative of timely, appropriate care with the managerial need to optimize resource use [39–41].

In this context, traditional triage systems focused solely on clinical priority revealed their limitations. Systems such as CTAS or ATS, although clinically sound, did not provide sufficient information for efficient flow management and resource allocation. The need for a more sophisticated approach that integrated clinical and managerial considerations into a single operational tool became evident.

The ESI project originated from collaboration between clinicians and researchers from several U.S. institutions, initially coordinated by the University of Pittsburgh and later further developed by a team led by the University of North Carolina [39].

The key conceptual innovation was the introduction of "resource intensity" as a dimension complementary to clinical acuity [39]. This idea arose from the observation that patients with the same clinical priority could have very different care needs in terms of diagnostic tests, treatments, and staff time.

Version 1 of the ESI, published in 1999, represented the first systematic attempt to build a decision algorithm integrating clinical acuity and resource prediction [39]. However, early experience quickly revealed some limitations, particularly in defining criteria for intermediate levels and in standardizing how resources were counted.

Version 2, released in 2003, introduced important refinements based on operational feedback and validation study results [40]. Major changes concerned simplification of the decision algorithm, clearer definitions of "danger zone vital signs," and more specific criteria for clinical risk assessment [40]. This version began to gain broad acceptance across U.S. emergency departments.

Version 3, published in 2005, was a smaller but significant revision that further refined operational criteria and introduced more detailed guidance for staff training [41]. It benefited from a large validation database that included data from hundreds of thousands of patients in diverse settings [41].

Version 4, released in 2012, represented the most substantial update since the original [39]. Key changes involved updating danger zone vital signs based on new evidence and introducing more specific criteria for special populations.

The latest version, Version 5 (2020), incorporated lessons learned during the COVID-19 pandemic and updates derived from two decades of operational experience and clinical research [42]. The revisions mainly refined risk criteria, updated guidance for managing infectious emergencies, and enhanced integration with modern digital technologies [42].

The evolution of the ESI has been supported by the Agency for Healthcare Research and Quality (AHRQ), which recognized its potential to improve the quality and efficiency of emergency care [39]. This institutional support facilitated widespread dissemination and provided resources for ongoing research and development.

4.3.3   System Objectives

The ESI was conceived with multidimensional objectives reflecting the complexity of challenges faced by modern EDs. Unlike more traditional triage systems focused mainly on clinical prioritization, the ESI pursues an integrated vision that combines patient safety, operational efficiency, and resource optimization within a coherent, practical framework.

The primary objective of the ESI is to ensure that the most critical patients receive immediate attention by rapidly and accurately identifying conditions requiring life-saving interventions or carrying a high risk of deterioration [39, 42]. This goal is achieved through the first two levels of the system (ESI 1 and ESI 2), which are designed to maximize sensitivity for true emergencies, even at the expense of lower specificity. The underlying philosophy is that no critically ill patient should be underestimated and that false positives in these categories are clinically and legally preferable to false negatives [39, 42].

A second key objective is optimization of resource allocation through accurate prediction of diagnostic and therapeutic resource use [39, 42]. This conceptual innovation distinguishes the ESI from all previous triage systems and addresses a concrete operational need: in modern EDs, efficiency depends not only on the speed of patient assessment but also on the ability to direct patients to the most appropriate care pathways based on the complexity of their needs.

Resource prediction also facilitates appropriate staffing and operational planning. Knowing in advance that a patient will likely require multiple diagnostic investigations, specialist consultations, or complex treatments allows for proactive resource allocation and helps prevent bottlenecks that could compromise the efficiency of the entire system [39, 42].

Finally, the ESI aims to be economically sustainable by contributing to cost control through more efficient use of diagnostic and therapeutic resources. The ability to predict resource consumption enables more accurate planning and can reduce waste associated with over-investigation or under-investigation.

4.3.4   Clinical Functioning of the System

The ESI is characterized by a decision architecture that is simple yet conceptually sophisticated, combining assessment of clinical acuity with prediction of resource use through a linear algorithm based on binary questions [39, 42]. This structure allows the triage nurse to progress rapidly through the decision process, minimizing operational complexity while maintaining high accuracy in patient classification.

The ESI is organized as a hierarchical decision tree with four main decision points, each of which can directly determine the final priority level or lead to the next step. This hierarchy ensures that the most critical conditions are identified immediately, while stable patients are classified according to the expected complexity of their care.

The operational philosophy of the ESI is based on a "worst-case scenario" principle: when doubt exists about the appropriate category, the system is designed to favor the more conservative choice from a clinical standpoint [39, 42]. This reflects the absolute priority given to patient safety over operational efficiency, while still maintaining a balance that avoids systematic over-triage.

A distinctive feature of the ESI is the integration of objective physiological criteria (danger zone vital signs) with subjective clinical assessments (high-risk conditions, severe pain, or distress). This combination allows the system to capture both conditions with obvious vital sign abnormalities and those that, despite normal or only mildly altered parameters, carry substantial clinical risk.

The system incorporates multiple safeguards to reduce the risk of under-triage. Danger zone vital signs function as an automatic "safety net," while subjective assessment of clinical risk enables experienced triage nurses to detect conditions that may not be immediately apparent from objective parameters alone [39, 42].

4.3.5   Acuity Levels

The ESI employs a five-level structure that reflects its dual philosophy, differentiating clearly between levels based on clinical acuity (ESI 1–2) and levels based on care complexity (ESI 3–5). Understanding this conceptual distinction is essential to grasp the operational logic of the system and its organizational implications.

ESI 1 (Resuscitation): Maximum priority, including patients requiring immediate life-saving interventions. This category is reserved for conditions with imminent threat to life that tolerate no delay. The assignment of ESI 1 triggers immediate activation of the resuscitation team and direct transfer to the resuscitation area. Target time: absolute immediacy (0 minutes) [42].

ESI 2 (Emergent): Includes high-risk patients or those with danger zone vital signs. This category embodies the main ESI innovation for high-priority patients, combining manifest physiological instability with conditions at high risk of rapid deterioration, even when currently stable. The suggested time target is within approximately 15 minutes, though emphasis is placed on prompt assessment rather than strict adherence to a fixed time threshold [42].

ESI 3 (Urgent): A transitional level where the ESI shifts from a purely clinical logic to integration of operational considerations. ESI 3 patients are clinically stable but expected to require two or more types of resources to reach a disposition decision (discharge or admission). Typical examples include patients with acute but stable conditions requiring complex diagnostic work-ups, such as abdominal pain requiring both laboratory tests and imaging [42].

ESI 4 (Less Urgent): Stable patients expected to need only one type of resource. This category includes relatively simple conditions requiring a single diagnostic or therapeutic intervention, such as a patient with an uncomplicated laceration requiring suturing only [42].

ESI 5 (Nonurgent): Patients who are not expected to require hospital resources to resolve their problem. This includes very minor conditions, prescription renewals, routine checks, and administrative issues [42].

The distinction between ESI 3, 4, and 5 based on the number of resource types required is the most innovative aspect of the system, enabling accurate prediction of care complexity and facilitating internal flow management in the ED [42].

4.3.6 How the Acuity Level Is Assigned

Assignment of the ESI level follows a structured sequence of four main decision points, each formulated as a binary question that guides the triage nurse toward the appropriate classification.

1. First decision point: Does the patient require immediate life-saving interventions?

   The process always begins by assessing whether life-saving interventions are required. This question is designed to instantly identify conditions that need immediate resuscitation. Criteria for a "yes" answer include: airway compromise requiring immediate intervention; absent or inadequate breathing requiring ventilatory support; absent or non-palpable pulse; shock with severe hemodynamic instability; severely impaired level of consciousness (GCS $\leq$ 8); ongoing seizures; major trauma with multi-organ instability.

   A positive response leads to the immediate assignment of ESI 1 and activation of the resuscitation team. This assessment must be completed within the first 30 seconds and does not require formal measurement of vital signs.

2. Second decision point: Is the patient high risk, confused/lethargic, in severe pain/distress, or presenting danger zone vital signs?

   If the patient does not require immediate life-saving interventions, a more detailed assessment follows, integrating different dimensions of risk:

   I. High-risk conditions: Conditions that, although not requiring immediate resuscitation, carry high evolution potential or are time-sensitive. Examples include chest pain suggestive of acute coronary syndrome, new-onset acute dyspnea, acute focal neurological deficits, and significant active bleeding.

  II. Altered mental status: Acute changes in mental state, confusion, lethargy, or major behavioral changes relative to baseline.

 III. Severe pain or distress: Severe pain (typically >7/10 on a numerical rating scale) or substantial distress that compromises the patient's ability to wait without intervention.

 IV. Danger zone vital signs: The most objective component of ESI level-2 assessment. The presence of any altered vital signs leads to assignment of ESI 2. Danger zone vital signs are intentionally calibrated to favor sensitivity over specificity, functioning as a safety net for potentially critical conditions.

3. Third decision point: How many resources will be required?

   For patients who do not meet criteria for ESI 1 or 2, classification is based on predicting the number of resource types likely needed to reach a disposition decision.

   Resources are counted by type, not by number of tests, and include, for example, laboratory tests, imaging studies, ECG, procedures (e.g., suturing, fracture reduction), specialist consultations, and IV fluids or medications.

   Resource counting is based on a reasonable prediction of what will be required, not on rigid protocols. The triage nurse uses clinical judgement to estimate needs based on the presenting complaint and experience.

4. Fourth decision point: Final assignment

   Based on the resource prediction: ≥ 2 resource types equal to ESI 3; 1 resource type equal to ESI 4; 0 resources equal to ESI 5.

The ESI also foresees special situations that may modify the standard assignment. The system preserves flexibility for justified clinical override, acknowledging that complex situations may not be fully captured by the standard algorithm. Any override must be clearly documented to enable audit and continuous improvement [39, 42].

4.3.7   Development and Internal Validation

The ESI is a paradigmatic example of how translational research can generate innovative clinical tools by systematically integrating scientific evidence, clinical experience, and principles of operations engineering. Its development followed a rigorous methodology combining large-scale retrospective analyses, prospective validation studies, and real-world operational testing, resulting in a system that is both scientifically sound and practically feasible [43].

The development process began with an in-depth analysis of limitations of existing triage systems. The foundational phase consisted of a retrospective analysis of

ED visits across several U.S. hospitals. The objective was to identify predictive patterns linking presenting characteristics with clinical outcomes and resource use. Researchers systematically examined the relationships among arrival vital signs, presenting complaints, diagnostic and therapeutic interventions, length of stay, need for admission, mortality, and costs.

A crucial methodological innovation was the introduction of "resource intensity" as a quantifiable, predictive dimension. Researchers developed a taxonomy of hospital resources, categorized by type rather than volume, and demonstrated that the number of resource types used correlated strongly with care complexity, length of stay, and costs. This finding provided the empirical basis for the dual architecture of the ESI: clinical acuity for higher levels and resource prediction for lower levels.

Definition of danger zone vital signs was another critical component. Researchers analyzed vital sign distributions in relation to adverse outcomes, identifying thresholds that maximized sensitivity for critical conditions while maintaining acceptable specificity.

Internal validation of the ESI was conducted through a structured research program including several study types. Construct validity was tested by assessing correlations between ESI levels and predefined clinical outcomes.

Inter-rater reliability studies using both real patients and standardized scenarios reported weighted kappa coefficients around 0.791, with highest agreement for extreme levels (ESI 1 and 5) and greater variability for intermediate levels [43–46]. These results were considered satisfactory and comparable to other validated triage systems.

Results confirmed that the ESI could be effectively implemented in diverse settings while maintaining satisfactory performance [43, 46, 47].

An innovative aspect of internal validation was the focus on economic evaluation. Cost-effectiveness studies showed that ESI implementation generated significant savings by reducing length of stay, optimizing diagnostic resource use, and decreasing readmissions [48].

Development of the ESI also included creation of a comprehensive implementation ecosystem: detailed operational manuals, structured training materials, case-based teaching tools, and audit and quality-monitoring instruments [39, 42]. This systemic approach was essential to ensure effective implementation and sustained quality over time.

4.3.8 External Validation

Following its official introduction in 1999, the ESI underwent extensive external validation across hundreds of healthcare facilities in the United States and internationally. This process is one of the most comprehensive ever conducted for a triage system and has produced a substantial evidence base confirming its scientific credibility and clarifying conditions for optimal implementation.

Initial external validation studies were conducted in U.S. emergency departments with characteristics different from those used in system development.

Interrater reliability varies substantially across studies depending on methodology, population, and rater experience. A meta-analysis of 19 studies reported a pooled reliability coefficient of 0.791 (95% CI 0.787–0.795), indicating substantial agreement overall. Scenario-based studies typically report higher reliability (weighted kappa 0.77–0.89), while real-patient assessments show more variability, with weighted kappas ranging from 0.57 to 0.75 [43–47]. Agreement tends to be highest for extreme acuity levels (ESI 1 and 5) and more variable for intermediate levels (ESI 2 and 3).

Pediatric validation was a major focus, as the system was originally developed for adults. Studies in pediatric EDs showed that ESI maintains good performance in children, with adjusted danger zone vital signs reflecting pediatric physiology [45, 49].

International validation began in the 2000s, with studies from Switzerland, the UK, and several European countries confirming that ESI retained its performance characteristics in health systems organized differently from the U.S. These studies also highlighted the need for local adaptations, particularly in resource definitions and care pathways [47, 50, 51].

4.3.9   Role of the Triage Nurse

Within the ESI system, the triage nurse plays a strategic, multidimensional role that reflects both the conceptual sophistication of the tool and the complex operational demands of modern EDs [39, 42]. Unlike more traditional triage systems, where the nurse mainly applies clinical criteria, in the ESI the professional must integrate clinical assessment, operational prediction, and strategic decision-making, becoming a key player in optimizing patient flow.

Selection of triage nurses for ESI use follows specific criteria reflecting system complexity. Candidates must also possess strong clinical judgment, multitasking ability, and an aptitude for analytical thinking required for resource prediction.

Standard training programs usually include a didactic phase covering theoretical foundations, the decision algorithm, danger zone vital signs, high-risk criteria and, crucially, methods for resource prediction [39, 42]. This is followed by hours of supervised practical training, during which the candidate applies the ESI under the guidance of an experienced mentor [39, 42].

A distinctive feature of ESI training is the emphasis on resource prediction, which requires a deep understanding of diagnostic and therapeutic pathways and ED operational dynamics. The nurse must develop the ability to "look ahead" along the patient pathway, anticipating which investigations, consultations, and treatments will likely be required based on the initial presentation [52]. This predictive capability is central to the system's operational effectiveness and demands experience and ongoing education.

Technical competencies include full command of the decision algorithm, from assessing the need for life-saving interventions to accurately predicting resource use [39, 42, 53]. The nurse must be able to measure and interpret vital signs, recognize danger zone vital signs, identify high-risk conditions, evaluate pain and distress intensity, and develop structured clinical reasoning to estimate resource requirements.

The role also includes significant educational and mentoring responsibilities toward less experienced colleagues. In departments using the ESI, the expert triage nurse serves as a reference for practical training, management of complex cases, and maintenance of quality standards.

Documentation responsibilities are substantial. The nurse must record the reasoning underlying the assigned level, particularly for ESI 2 patients, where subjective risk assessment is crucial, and, for ESI 3–5, must document predicted resources and the rationale. These data are essential for clinical audit and continuous improvement.

Finally, the ESI triage nurse has a strategic role in optimizing operational flow. Accurate resource prediction directly influences departmental efficiency, space utilization, staff allocation, and patient satisfaction. This strategic responsibility requires an overall understanding of ED dynamics and the ability to balance individual patient needs with system-wide efficiency.

4.3.10 Special Populations

The maturity and completeness of the ESI are evident in the attention devoted to special populations, acknowledging that different patient groups require tailored assessment approaches while preserving coherence with the system's core architecture. This adaptability is one of the most important evolutionary aspects of the ESI and reflects its application in increasingly diverse, complex clinical settings.

Adapting the ESI to children posed major challenges and required substantial modifications reflecting physiological, anatomical, and behavioral differences. The Pediatric Emergency Severity Index (Ped-ESI) maintains the four-step decision structure of the adult system but introduces age-specific vital signs and adapted criteria for different age ranges [45, 54].

Pediatric danger zone vital signs are stratified by age, acknowledging marked variations in normal values from birth to adolescence [45, 54].

A distinctive element is the use of behavioral and social interaction criteria as severity indicators. Inconsolable irritability, reduced social responsiveness, altered feeding patterns, and inappropriate lethargy are considered equivalent to danger zone vital signs for assignment of ESI 2, recognizing that in young children signs of clinical compromise often manifest as behavioral change before vital-sign instability [54, 55].

Pain assessment uses age-appropriate scales: FLACC for nonverbal children, numeric scales for verbal children, and behavioral tools for those with cognitive impairment. Severe pain (>7/10 or behavioral equivalent) remains relevant for the ESI 2 assignment but requires specific pediatric assessment expertise.

Management of pregnant patients in the ESI requires considerations that encompass both maternal and fetal well-being, physiological changes of pregnancy, and specific obstetric emergencies requiring urgent intervention [42].

Danger zone vital signs are adapted to pregnancy physiology. Mild tachycardia and positional hypotension are common in late pregnancy, while even moderate hypertension may indicate pre-eclampsia and require urgent evaluation. Fever has lower thresholds for concern, particularly in the first trimester and peripartum [42].

Obstetric conditions that automatically trigger ESI 2 include significant vaginal bleeding at any gestational age, severe abdominal pain with suspected ectopic pregnancy, signs of pre-eclampsia/eclampsia, preterm labor, premature rupture of membranes, and marked reduction in fetal movements after 20 weeks [42].

4.3.11 Strengths and Clinical Advantages

The ESI has several strengths that have made it one of the most widely used and appreciated triage systems worldwide [42]. Its advantages stem from its unique conceptual architecture, operational simplicity, and integrated approach combining clinical and managerial considerations.

The main strength is its core conceptual innovation: integrating assessment of clinical acuity with prediction of resource use. This distinguishes ESI from all preceding triage systems and meets a concrete operational need in modern emergency departments. While traditional systems simply rank patients by urgency, ESI simultaneously provides crucial information for flow management and resource allocation.

This duality supports more sophisticated patient management, enabling differentiated care pathways based not only on severity but also on complexity. ESI 4–5 patients can be managed efficiently in areas by less specialized staff, whereas ESI 3 patients can be directed to intermediate-intensity zones with appropriate diagnostic capabilities. This organization optimizes use of space and personnel, improving overall efficiency.

The decision architecture, based on four sequential binary questions, is a model of operational elegance, combining clinical completeness and rapid application. Triage nurses can navigate the algorithm within minutes, often reaching a decision before completing all steps. This speed is crucial in high-volume settings where triage time must be minimized to avoid bottlenecks.

Algorithm linearity significantly reduces the risk of procedural errors and facilitates memorization. Unlike more complex systems requiring frequent consultation of manuals or tables, ESI can be applied entirely from memory after appropriate training, increasing speed and fluidity of the process.

Another strength is the breadth of its scientific validation. Hundreds of peer-reviewed studies have confirmed its validity, reliability, and operational utility in various contexts [1, 2]. Evidence encompasses not only traditional clinical outcomes (mortality, admission, and length of stay) but also innovative managerial metrics such as resource consumption, operational efficiency, and staff and patient satisfaction.

4.3.12 Critical Issues and Clinical Limitations

Despite its many strengths and broad international acceptance, the ESI presents limitations and critical aspects that must be recognized and managed appropriately to optimize effectiveness. These do not necessarily undermine overall utility but require awareness and targeted mitigation strategies to minimize impact on safety and efficiency.

ESI effectiveness depends heavily on the quality of staff training and ongoing maintenance of competencies, particularly regarding assessment of high-risk conditions and resource prediction. Unlike danger zone vital signs, which are objective and easy to verify, these elements require sophisticated clinical judgment and consolidated experience.

Assessment of high-risk conditions is one of the system's most vulnerable points. Recognizing that a patient with atypical chest pain may have acute coronary syndrome, or that a patient with mild dyspnea may have pulmonary embolism, demands expertise and knowledge that not all triage nurses possess. This variability can lead to significant differences in system performance between operators [43].

Resource prediction, the ESI's innovative hallmark, poses particular challenges. It requires deep understanding of diagnostic-therapeutic pathways, indications for investigations, and ED operational dynamics. This competence develops through experience and is difficult to standardize solely through theoretical training.

Although resource prediction is a strength, it is also a major source of complexity and potential error. Accurate estimation of resource types requires understanding not only the patient's condition but also local diagnostic protocols, physician preferences, and specific departmental workflows. The very definition of what constitutes a "resource" may vary between operators or institutions [43].

Resource prediction is also influenced by extrinsic factors such as imaging availability, consultation response times, and hospital admission policies, which can render an initially correct prediction inaccurate. Variability in clinical practice among physicians further complicates standardization.

Moreover, continuous evolution in medical practice, the introduction of new diagnostic technologies, and epidemiological changes require periodic updates to ESI to preserve accuracy and relevance. Validating such updates demands large, costly, and time-consuming studies.

At the same time, growing clinical complexity and rising expectations have increased overall resource use, even for ruling out severe or time-sensitive conditions. Compared with the 1990s, many diagnostic tools, especially laboratory tests and CT imaging, are now more accessible and frequently used. Since the ESI uses the number of resources as a key determinant of triage level, this general increase in resource use directly affects urgency assignment, potentially shifting more patients into higher levels.

Balancing system stability with the need for continuous updating is therefore a constant challenge: overly frequent modifications risk undermining standardization, whereas infrequent revisions may render the system obsolete.

4.4 Manchester Triage System MTS

4.4.1 Introduction

The Manchester Triage System (MTS) is one of the most significant developments in the European landscape of triage systems, distinguished by a rigorous methodological approach that places standardization, reproducibility, and auditability at the center of its design [1, 2]. Developed in the late 1990s in the United Kingdom, the MTS revolutionized hospital triage by introducing a structured methodology based on presentation flowcharts that explicitly and transparently link the patient's presenting complaint to the priority level assigned [56].

The fundamental philosophy of the MTS rests on a principle of decision-making transparency that clearly differentiates it from many contemporary triage systems [56]. While numerous systems rely on general algorithms or global parametric assessments, the MTS adopts a granular approach that breaks the decision-making process down into explicit, verifiable steps, creating a system that is at once clinically robust and methodologically transparent [56].

The architecture of the MTS is built around the concept of a specific presenting complaint, with more than fifty dedicated flowcharts covering virtually all clinical presentations seen in emergency departments [56]. This specificity is both the main strength of the system, its ability to provide detailed guidance for each type of presentation, and one of its operational challenges, namely the need to master a large number of distinct decision pathways [56].

The MTS also introduced the concept of "secondary triage" and dynamic reassessment as integral components of the system, recognizing that triage is not a single event but a continuous process that must adapt to changes in the patient's clinical condition [56]. This dynamic vision has had a major influence on the subsequent development of international triage systems, shifting the focus from simple initial classification to continuous risk management.

The diffusion of the MTS across Europe has been facilitated by its ability to adapt to different national health-care contexts while preserving methodological coherence [57, 58]. Countries such as Germany, Sweden, Italy, and many others have adopted the MTS with local adaptations, creating a network of implementations that has contributed to its large-scale validation and ongoing refinement [57, 59, 60].

The impact of the MTS extends beyond the purely clinical sphere and has significantly influenced the culture of quality and audit within European EDs. Its emphasis on structured documentation and process measurability has helped raise standards of clinical governance and has provided concrete tools for the continuous improvement of emergency care quality.

4.4.2 History: Origins, Context of Development and Evolution

The MTS emerged during a period of profound transformation in the British healthcare system, characterized by reforms introduced by the Conservative governments of the 1980s and 1990s and by a growing emphasis on quality, efficiency, and accountability in health services [56]. The National Health Service (NHS) was undergoing restructuring, with the introduction of the internal market, explicit performance standards, and a culture of audit that required objective measurement tools for evaluating the quality of care.

The specific context that led to the birth of the MTS was marked by increasing pressure on British EDs. The 1990s saw a constant rise in ED attendances, the introduction of government targets for waiting times, and increasing media and political scrutiny of emergency care performance. In this setting, the absence of standardized triage systems represented a major problem for clinical governance and quality monitoring.

Before the introduction of the MTS, British EDs used heterogeneous triage systems, often based on local protocols or on adaptations of international tools that had not been validated in the NHS context. This fragmentation made benchmarking between hospitals impossible and undermined the system's capacity to monitor and systematically improve the quality of care.

The initiative that led to the development of the MTS originated at Manchester Royal Infirmary, where a multidisciplinary group of clinicians began working on a triage system tailored to the specific needs of the British context [56]. The group included emergency physicians, specialist nurses, quality and safety experts, and representatives of national professional organizations.

The development methodology was innovative for its time, using a systematic approach that combined international literature review, analysis of clinical databases, consensus development, and operational testing in real-world settings [56]. The working group analyzed thousands of clinical cases in order to identify the most common presenting complaints and to develop discriminators that best predicted clinical urgency and adverse outcomes.

A distinctive feature of the MTS development process was the emphasis placed from the outset on validation and audit. The system was designed not only to be clinically accurate but also to be readily auditable and subject to improvement through systematic feedback [56]. This philosophy reflected the emerging NHS culture centered on evidence-based practice and continuous quality improvement.

The first version of the MTS was published in 1997 and was quickly followed by a series of pilot studies in various hospitals in the North of England. Initial results were encouraging, showing good correlation between assigned priority and clinical outcomes and a marked reduction in inter-observer variability compared with previous systems.

This initial success led to the formal adoption of the MTS by the Manchester Triage Group, a consortium of hospitals and professional organizations that took responsibility for the system's development and dissemination. This organizational structure, unique in the triage landscape, provided dedicated resources for research, further development, and implementation support.

International expansion of the MTS began in the early 2000s, when several European countries started piloting the system. Germany was among the first to adopt the MTS on a large scale, followed by other nations [57–59]. Each national implementation involved specific adaptations to reflect local health-system characteristics, while preserving the core methodological structure.

The third version of the MTS, published in 2014, benefited from accumulated international experience and introduced further refinements based on over a decade of use in diverse settings [56]. Key changes involved updating the underlying evidence base, adding new flowcharts for emerging conditions, and improving integration with electronic health systems.

A crucial milestone was official recognition by the Royal College of Emergency Medicine and the Royal College of Nursing, which adopted the MTS as the recommended standard for triage in UK EDs. This endorsement greatly facilitated dissemination and secured resources for ongoing training and support.

The evolution of the MTS has also been characterized by the development of a comprehensive support ecosystem, including standardized training programs, operator certification systems, automated audit tools, and an international research network that continues to validate and refine the system.

4.4.3   System Objectives

The MTS was conceived with multidimensional objectives that reflect a sophisticated view of triage as a clinical, organizational and quality-management process. Unlike systems developed mainly to address immediate operational needs, the MTS was designed from the outset as an instrument for cultural and methodological transformation in emergency departments, with ambitions far beyond simple patient classification.

The primary objective of the MTS is to standardize the triage decision-making process by eliminating arbitrariness and uncontrolled subjectivity [56]. The system aims to create a common language and shared criteria that allow different professionals, in different hospitals and at different times, to reach consistent decisions when faced with similar clinical presentations. This standardization is not an end in itself; it is instrumental in improving patient safety and reducing inappropriate variability in care.

A second key objective is the creation of a fully auditable and transparent system [56]. The MTS is designed to make every step of the decision-making process explicit, from selection of the presentation flowchart to the choice of the final discriminator. This transparency serves multiple purposes: it facilitates clinical audit, allows identification of areas for improvement, supports staff training, and provides a solid basis for research and system development [56, 60].

The MTS also aims to raise the quality of clinical documentation in emergency departments. Through its mandatory structured documentation, the system ensures that critical information is systematically collected and recorded, thereby improving continuity of care and providing high-quality data for research and audit [60–62]. This focus on documentation reflects the NHS culture of evidence-based practice and professional accountability.

A distinctive objective of the MTS is the systematic integration of pain assessment and management into the triage process [56]. The system recognizes that pain is not just a symptom to be recorded but a central component of the patient's experience that requires specific attention and timely intervention. This philosophy has helped shift professional culture regarding pain management in European emergency departments.

The MTS is also designed to support dynamic reassessment and secondary triage as integral components of care [56]. The system recognizes that patients' conditions can change during waiting times and that initial triage must be continually re-evaluated and updated. This dynamic view has significantly influenced the development of monitoring and reassessment protocols in emergency departments.

Another strategic objective is to support clinical governance and continuous quality improvement. The MTS provides specific, standardized metrics that allow clinical managers to monitor performance, identify problematic trends, and implement improvement initiatives based on objective data [56]. This capacity to underpin governance has made the MTS particularly attractive for health systems that emphasize accountability and transparency.

The system also aims to facilitate training and professional development for triage staff. Its explicit structure and transparent methodology make the MTS an effective educational tool, enabling staff to develop triage competence within a structured, verifiable framework [56, 60, 63]. This educational role is supported by standardized training programs and certification systems that ensure uniform competency standards.

An often under-recognized but extremely important objective is the creation of a standardized database for clinical research. The widespread use of the MTS in Europe has generated homogeneous data sets that facilitate multicenter studies and meta-analyses, contributing to advances in emergency medicine science [62, 64].

The system is also intended to be economically sustainable, contributing to optimal resource use through better prioritization and reduced waste associated with inappropriate or redundant assessments.

4.4.4　Clinical Functioning of the System

The MTS is characterized by an operational architecture that combines methodological rigor with practical usability through a modular structure based on specific presentation flowcharts [56]. This architecture is unique among triage systems, privileging specificity of assessment over generic algorithms and producing a system that is granular in its application yet coherent in its methodology [56].

The MTS process always begins with the identification of the patient's main presenting complaint, which determines the selection of the appropriate flowchart from more than fifty available. This selection phase is crucial because it defines the entire subsequent assessment pathway and demands specific skills in determining the primary reason for attendance when patients present with multiple or complex symptoms.

Once the appropriate flowchart has been selected, the triage nurse proceeds through a structured sequence of discriminators organized in hierarchical order of urgency. Discriminators are specific clinical elements (signs, symptoms, situations) that, if present, automatically determine the priority level [56]. The fundamental principle is that the triage nurse must select the first applicable discriminator, proceeding from top to bottom, ensuring that the most urgent conditions are always identified first.

The system also incorporates a set of generic discriminators that apply across all clinical presentations. These cover vital functions (airway, breathing, circulation, neurological status) and constitute a safety net ensuring that critical conditions are recognized regardless of the specific flowchart.

A distinctive feature of the MTS is the systematic integration of pain assessment in each flowchart. Pain is not treated solely as a symptom but as an active discriminator capable of directly influencing the assigned priority. This integration reflects the system's philosophy that pain management is a key indicator of care quality [56].

The MTS also provides specific mechanisms for structured documentation of every decision made during the triage process. This documentation is not merely an administrative requirement but an active tool for audit, training, and continuous quality improvement.

4.4.5   Acuity Levels

The Manchester Triage System uses a five-level color-coded classification, each level associated with specific target times for medical assessment. This temporal structure is one of the system's most rigorous elements, providing explicit targets that function both as operational guidance and as performance monitoring tools [56].

RED (Immediate—Priority 1): Represents the highest level of urgency and requires immediate clinical care, with no acceptable delay. This category includes conditions with imminent threat to life requiring immediate intervention.

ORANGE (Very Urgent—Priority 2): Includes patients who must be assessed within 10 minutes of priority assignment. This category comprises severe or potentially unstable conditions that, although not requiring instantaneous intervention, cannot safely wait without a significant risk of deterioration.

YELLOW (Urgent—Priority 3): Target time of 60 minutes. Includes patients with acute conditions requiring timely medical assessment but who can wait up to 1 hour without significant risk of deterioration.

GREEN (Standard—Priority 4): Assessment within 120 minutes (2 hours). Includes patients whose conditions do require medical care but are not significantly urgent and can wait without risk of worsening. This category includes exacerbations of chronic conditions, minor complaints, mild pain, and requests for check-ups or certificates.

BLUE (Nonurgent—Priority 5): Target time of 240 minutes (4 hours). Represents very minor conditions or administrative issues that can safely wait up to 4 hours without clinical consequences.

These target times are not conceived as rigid maximum limits but as operational benchmarks that enable performance monitoring and identification of systemic issues.

4.4.6   How the Acuity Level Is Assigned

The assignment of priority within the MTS follows a structured, sequential methodology using specific flowcharts and standardized discriminators.

I. Identification of the Presenting Complaint: The process always begins with accurate identification of the patient's main presenting complaint. This stage requires specific skills in active listening and interpretation of reported symptoms, especially when the patient presents multiple problems or vague complaints. The triage nurse must identify the primary reason that brought the patient to the ED, which may not coincide with the most obvious symptom at the time of assessment.

   The MTS provides guidance for selecting the appropriate presenting complaint when multiple symptoms are present. In general, the most acute, severe, or worrying symptom from the patient's perspective is prioritized. In cases of doubt, the system recommends choosing the presenting complaint most likely to lead to the highest priority, following the principle of safety [56].

II. Selection of the Appropriate Flowchart: Once the presenting complaint has been identified, the triage nurse selects the corresponding flowchart from the repertoire of over fifty available. Each flowchart is designed to cover a wide range of related clinical presentations, and accurate selection is crucial for an effective process [56].

   MTS flowcharts cover virtually all common ED presentations: chest pain, dyspnea, abdominal pain, headache, and many others. Each flowchart has been developed on the basis of specific clinical evidence and validated in multicenter studies.

III. Application of General Discriminators: Before applying the flowchart's specific discriminators, the triage nurse must evaluate the general discriminators that apply across all presentations. These fundamental safety discriminators include: airway, breathing, shock (circulatory compromise), level of consciousness, severe pain, temperature, and hemorrhage.

The presence of any markedly abnormal general discriminator results in automatic assignment of a high priority (typically red or orange), regardless of the specific flowchart [56].

IV. Application of Flowchart-Specific Discriminators: If no general discriminator is present, the triage nurse proceeds with the sequential application of the flowchart's specific discriminators. These are organized hierarchically by urgency, from the most urgent (leading to red) to the least urgent (leading to blue).

The core principle is that the nurse must progress from top to bottom and select the first discriminator that fits the patient. This approach guarantees that highly urgent conditions are always recognized first and prevents under-triage due to overlooking high-priority discriminators.

V. Documentation and Finalization: Each decision made during triage must be documented in a structured manner. Documentation includes the identified presenting complaint, flowchart used, discriminator selected, assigned priority and rationale, pain assessment, and recorded vital signs [56].

VI. Secondary Triage and Re-assessment: The MTS emphasizes that triage is a dynamic process requiring ongoing re-assessment. Secondary triage may be necessary when the patient's condition changes during waiting, new information becomes available, initial interventions modify clinical presentation, or there is significant deterioration or improvement [56].

Reassessment follows the same methodology as the initial triage and may result in a change of priority. The system recommends reassessment intervals based on the initial priority: Orange patients every 15 minutes, yellow every 30 minutes, and green every 60 minutes.

The MTS decision-making process is designed to be both rigorous and flexible, providing a clear structure that supports, rather than replaces, clinical judgment. The combination of objective discriminators and subjective clinical assessment allows the system to capture both typical presentations and atypical or complex clinical situations.

4.4.7   Development and Internal Validation

The MTS is an exemplary case of applied clinical research producing operational tools through a rigorous methodology that integrates scientific evidence, professional consensus, and empirical validation. Its development was guided from the outset by evidence-based medicine principles and a philosophy of methodological transparency, making every stage of the process documented, verifiable, and replicable [56].

Development began with a systematic analysis of the limitations of existing triage systems and the specific needs of the British healthcare context. The Manchester

Triage Group conducted an extensive review of international triage literature, identifying the main gap as the lack of systems combining clinical accuracy, methodological reproducibility, and the capacity for systematic audit.

A crucial methodological innovation was the use of consensus development techniques to define discriminators.

A particularly innovative aspect was the development of a specific audit methodology. The system was designed to be fully auditable, with explicit criteria for assessing triage quality [56]. Key audit parameters included completeness of assessment, correct use of flowcharts, appropriateness of discriminator selection, accuracy of assigned priority, and inter-observer agreement.

Inter-observer reliability was assessed using a combination of real clinical cases and standardized scenarios. Initial studies reported weighted kappa coefficients between 0.65 and 0.85, with better performance for extreme levels (red and blue) and greater variability for intermediate levels [65–68].

Operational validation was conducted through pilot studies in hospitals with diverse profiles. These studies evaluated not only clinical accuracy but also operational feasibility, application times, staff acceptability, and impact on patient flow [62–64]. Results confirmed that, with adequate training and regular audit, the MTS could be effectively implemented in different settings while maintaining satisfactory clinical performance.

Development of the MTS was accompanied by the creation of a comprehensive implementation support ecosystem: detailed operational manuals for each flowchart, standardized training programs with certification, case banks for training, automated audit tools, and a support network for operational problem-solving [56].

4.4.8 External Validation

After its official introduction, the MTS underwent one of the most extensive external validation processes ever conducted for a triage system, involving hundreds of hospitals across multiple European countries and generating a substantial body of evidence that consolidated its credibility and supported ongoing improvement [62–64]. This validation has set methodological standards that continue to influence triage research.

Validation of the integrated audit methodology was particularly significant. A study examining implementation in Italian hospitals showed that systematic use of MTS audit tools led to progressive improvements in system performance over time [60, 63]. Hospitals performing regular audits demonstrated significant increases in triage accuracy and inter-observer agreement [60, 63].

International validation began in the early 2000s, with Germany among the first countries to conduct systematic studies on adaptation to its health-care context [57, 69, 70]. Pediatric validation was addressed in dedicated studies that confirmed effectiveness in children. A study published found that pediatric MTS sensitivity for ICU admission was 71% and specificity 85% [71].

4.4.9 Role of the Triage Nurse

Within the Manchester Triage System, the triage nurse plays a central, highly specialized role that goes far beyond the mechanical application of predefined criteria. It requires advanced clinical competence, structured decision-making skills, and sophisticated communication abilities [60, 72]. The MTS recognizes the nurse as an autonomous clinical professional capable of making complex decisions that directly influence patient safety and ED efficiency.

Selection of triage nurses under the MTS is governed by stringent criteria that reflect the system's complexity and the role's importance. Typically, 2–5 years of clinical experience in emergency or acute care are required, with demonstrated competence in rapid assessment of acutely ill patients and management of high-complexity situations.

MTS-specific training is among the most structured and rigorous in the triage field. The standard program developed by the Manchester Triage Group includes an intensive 24-hour theoretical component covering the system's foundations, flowchart methodology, use of discriminators, pain assessment, and principles of audit and quality assurance [56]. This is followed by hours of supervised practical training, during which candidates apply the MTS under the guidance of a certified mentor.

A distinctive aspect of MTS training is the emphasis on understanding system methodology rather than rote memorization of flowcharts. Nurses must develop a deep appreciation of the principles underlying system construction, the logic of discriminators, and the audit philosophy [56]. This methodological understanding is essential for correct application and for adapting to complex or atypical cases.

Technical competencies required of MTS nurses include full mastery of the more than fifty flowcharts, the ability to select the appropriate flowchart swiftly based on the presenting complaint, and skill in applying discriminators in the prescribed hierarchical sequence [56]. Nurses must also be proficient in pain assessment using appropriate scales for adults, children, and patients with cognitive impairment and in fulfilling the system's structured documentation requirements.

Management of general discriminators is another core responsibility. These cross-cutting discriminators require rapid, accurate evaluation of key vital functions. The nurse must recognize immediately any signs of airway compromise, respiratory distress, shock, significant neurological alteration, or other conditions warranting immediate high priority irrespective of the specific presenting complaint [56].

MTS nurses also have defined responsibilities in pain management that extend beyond assessment. Documentation in the MTS demands skills aligned with the system's emphasis on transparency and auditability. Nurses must record not only assessment findings but also the decision-making process: identified presenting complaint, flowchart used, discriminators evaluated, rationale for assigned priority, and any initial interventions. This detailed documentation is essential for clinical audits and medico-legal protection.

A distinctive aspect of the role is responsibility for secondary triage and dynamic reassessment [56]. Nurses must maintain active surveillance of waiting patients, periodically re-evaluating their condition and modifying priority as needed. This requires excellent organizational skills, attention to detail, and an ability to recognize clinically significant changes.

Finally, MTS nurses have specific responsibilities in audit and continuous quality improvement [60, 63, 72, 73]. They are expected to participate in audit programs, contribute to identifying systemic problems, and propose improvements based on operational experience, reflecting the MTS philosophy that every user is an active contributor to system refinement.

4.4.10 Special Populations

The MTS demonstrates its maturity and completeness through specific attention to populations requiring adapted assessment approaches, while maintaining the system's fundamental methodological coherence and recognizing the clinical, physiological, and social particularities of different patient groups. This specialized adaptability is one of the system's most significant evolutions.

Adapting the MTS to pediatrics has been one of the most complex and innovative challenges, requiring not only adjustment of physiological parameters but also a fundamental rethinking of certain assessment approaches to reflect the specificities of pediatric emergency medicine [74].

The pediatric MTS maintains the same methodological architecture as the adult version, with flowcharts for presenting complaints and hierarchical discriminators, but introduces substantial modifications reflecting pediatric physiology and disease presentation. Pediatric flowcharts were developed recognizing that many acute conditions in children manifest differently from adults and that children have compensatory mechanisms that may mask severity until advanced stages [56].

Pediatric general discriminators include age-specific vital sign ranges reflecting normal physiological variation from birth to adolescence [74, 75].

A distinctive element of pediatric MTS is the introduction of behavioral and social-interaction discriminators. Inconsolable irritability, reduced social responsiveness, altered feeding patterns, age-inappropriate lethargy, and abnormal cry quality are active discriminators that may justify high priority even when vital signs are apparently normal [56, 74, 75]. These recognize that, especially in young children, early signs of serious illness often manifest as behavioral changes before physiological instability becomes evident.

Pediatric pain assessment uses age-appropriate, culturally sensitive tools: behavioral scales such as FLACC for infants and neonates; pictorial scales such as Wong–Baker FACES for preschool children; and numerical scales for older children, with appropriate communication adaptations [56].

Pediatric-specific flowcharts address common presentations in children: fever in young infants, feeding difficulties, vomiting and diarrhea, rashes, pediatric respiratory problems, and pediatric trauma [56]. Each considers pediatric epidemiology and age-appropriate thresholds for concern.

A crucial aspect is the integration of parental or caregiver input into assessment. Parents are recognized as primary informants about deviations from the child's baseline, and their concerns are treated as active discriminators. The "parental concern" discriminator may increase priority even when objective parameters do not indicate high urgency [56].

Obstetric MTS content includes flowcharts for vaginal bleeding in pregnancy, abdominal pain in pregnancy, labor, and delivery, postpartum complications, and gynecological emergencies [56]. Each flowchart reflects the physiological and pathological characteristics of pregnancy and the reproductive cycle.

Obstetric discriminators interpret vital signs in light of normal pregnancy physiology. Mild tachycardia and positional hypotension are common in late pregnancy and do not automatically indicate high priority, whereas even moderate hypertension may signal pre-eclampsia and warrants urgent evaluation [56].

Specific obstetric conditions that automatically result in high priority include significant vaginal bleeding in any trimester, severe abdominal pain with suspected ectopic pregnancy, signs of pre-eclampsia/eclampsia (hypertension, proteinuria, headache, visual disturbance), preterm labor before 37 weeks, premature rupture of membranes, and marked reduction in fetal movements after 28 weeks [56].

Where appropriate and feasible, obstetric MTS integrates assessment of fetal well-being into triage, including evaluation of active movements and abnormal vaginal loss, all of which may directly influence assigned priority.

4.4.11 Strengths and Clinical Advantages

The MTS has numerous distinctive strengths that have made it one of the most respected and widely used triage systems internationally, particularly in European EDs [1, 2, 62, 64]. These advantages derive from its rigorous methodological architecture, its defining transparency, and its systematic approach to quality and continuous improvement.

The MTS excels in standardizing the triage process, markedly reducing interoperator variability typical of less structured systems [67]. Presenting-complaint-specific flowcharts eliminate much of the arbitrariness of initial assessment, while hierarchical discriminators ensure that urgent conditions are always considered first.

This standardization is particularly important in settings with staff of heterogeneous experience and training. A relatively inexperienced nurse, if following MTS flowcharts correctly, can reach decisions consistent with those of more senior colleagues. This is crucial for system safety and for large-scale implementation.

Reduced variability has major implications for research and benchmarking. Data generated by hospitals using MTS are comparable and can be pooled for multicenter studies, meta-analyses, and performance comparisons between institutions [72, 73]. This comparability has significantly advanced knowledge in triage and emergency medicine.

The MTS was designed from inception with integrated audit methodology that is a benchmark in triage. Audit tools allow systematic evaluation of triage quality through specific, measurable indicators such as completeness of assessment, correct flowchart usage, appropriateness of discriminator selection, accuracy of assigned priority, and inter-observer agreement [60, 63].

This audit capability has transformed quality culture in European EDs: hospitals using MTS can continuously monitor performance, identify problematic trends, and implement data-driven improvement actions. Benchmarking between institutions and identification of best practices are facilitated, and hospitals with superior performance can disseminate their strategies, enhancing system-wide quality [60, 63, 72, 76].

The scientific foundations of the MTS are robust, with each discriminator based on specific clinical evidence and empirically validated. The development methodology, combining consensus development techniques, clinical database analysis, and empirical validation, provides a model for evidence-based clinical tool development and underpins the system's credibility.

The MTS continues to evolve in response to new scientific evidence through periodic revisions that incorporate current research findings, ensuring that the system remains clinically relevant and up to date.

4.4.12 Limitations and Clinical Disadvantages

Despite its many strengths and wide acceptance in the European clinical community, the MTS has limitations and critical points that must be recognized and managed to optimize effectiveness and minimize potential risks. These limitations do not negate the system's overall utility but require awareness and targeted mitigation strategies.

One major limitation is inherent operational complexity, stemming from the need to master more than fifty flowcharts and hundreds of specific discriminators. This complexity, although the source of the system's specificity and accuracy, can constitute a significant barrier to implementation and to maintaining optimal performance.

The learning curve for MTS is considerably steeper than for simpler systems. Staff must not only become familiar with numerous flowcharts but also develop competence in rapidly selecting the appropriate one based on the presenting complaint and navigating the hierarchical discriminators. This demands substantial investment in initial and ongoing training [72, 73].

System complexity can contribute to operational errors when staff are under pressure or inadequately trained [76]. Incorrect flowchart selection, failure to follow the hierarchical sequence of discriminators, or misinterpretation of specific criteria can compromise accuracy [63]. These errors are more likely in early implementation phases or where staff turnover is high.

In settings with limited training resources or high reliance on temporary staff, MTS complexity may significantly hinder effective use.

System effectiveness depends critically on the quality of initial training and maintenance of competence [72, 73]. Unlike simpler systems that can be applied with minimal training, MTS requires deep methodological understanding, flowchart mastery, and structured clinical reasoning skills. Variability in training quality can lead to marked differences in performance between staff and across institutions.

Compliance with MTS methodology is another challenge. The system requires strict adherence: always using the appropriate flowchart, applying discriminators in hierarchical order, and documenting the decision process. Deviations, even when motivated by clinical good intentions, can undermine accuracy, reproducibility, and auditability.

Maintaining compliance over time necessitates regular audits, systematic feedback, and refresher training programs. Without these supports, MTS performance tends to deteriorate, with increased inter-operator variability and reduced decision accuracy [63].

The MTS also embodies an intrinsic tension between the methodological rigidity needed for standardization and reproducibility and the clinical flexibility required to manage real-world complexity and variability. This can create operational challenges: rigid adherence may be perceived as restrictive by experienced clinicians, while excessive flexibility can erode the very benefits of standardization.

Although the system allows clinical override, it's appropriate use requires highly developed clinical judgement and may itself become a source of variability if not well regulated. Documentation of overrides is essential but may be perceived as time-consuming and bureaucratic.

In summary, the MTS is a powerful, scientifically grounded, and highly standardized triage tool whose benefits are maximized when supported by robust training, strong organizational commitment to audit and quality, and a careful balance between methodological fidelity and clinical judgment.

4.5   Canadian Triage and Acuity Scale

4.5.1   Introduction

The Canadian Triage and Acuity Scale (CTAS) is now one of the most widely used and internationally recognized triage systems [77]. Developed in Canada in the 1990s, it has been the subject of numerous studies and successive updates that have consolidated its validity and supported its continuous evolution [77].

Over time, CTAS has crossed national borders, being implemented in multiple countries, translated into several languages, and adapted to different healthcare settings [78, 79]. Initially conceived for hospital emergency departments, it has progressively been extended to the pre-hospital environment as well, becoming a reference tool both for day-to-day ED operations and for the planning of complex emergency care systems [80, 81].

Its design aimed to address the fragmentation of access to Canadian EDs by standardizing the assessment of patients presenting in emergency and quantifying clinical severity in a reproducible way. Marked variability between hospitals and professionals was generating significant differences in waiting times, resource allocation, and, ultimately, patient safety [82].

CTAS introduced a structured, evidence-based approach that stratifies patients into five priority levels, from most critical to least urgent [77, 83]. The fundamental principle is that access to care should not depend on order of arrival but on clinical urgency and the potential risk of deterioration [77, 83]. Each level is associated with a target time for physician assessment, which promotes equity of access and allows continuous monitoring of service quality.

A distinctive feature of CTAS is its close link with the Canadian Emergency Department Information System (CEDIS), a standardized list of presenting complaints that helps clinicians classify patients consistently [84]. The use of objective criteria, such as vital signs, pain intensity, and mechanism of injury, has improved the reliability of the system and facilitated its scientific validation [77, 83].

Over time, CTAS has undergone several revisions to refine the definition of levels and introduce specific modifiers for particular populations, such as children and patients with psychiatric disorders [73, 83, 85, 86]. Its adoption is now widespread across Canada and has influenced triage models in many other countries, confirming its role not only as a clinical tool but also as an organizational and managerial reference for emergency care.

4.5.2   History: Origin, Context of Development, and Evolution

CTAS emerged in Canada in a healthcare system that, in the 1990s, was founded on the principle of universal public health coverage, guaranteeing free hospital care for all citizens. While this model represented a cornerstone of social equity, it began to show signs of considerable strain.

A steady increase in demand for care, progressive growth in ED attendances, population aging, inequities between urban and rural areas, and reductions in available resources were all undermining the system's ability to provide uniform and timely care.

Before CTAS was introduced, Canadian EDs were characterized by substantial organizational fragmentation: there was no single reference system, and each hospital applied its own criteria, often based on the individual experience of staff. This led to considerable variability in priority assignment, with consequences for waiting times, resource distribution, and patient safety. The situation was even more complex in rural and remote areas, where smaller hospitals operated with very limited resources.

In 1998, a multidisciplinary group of emergency physicians and triage nurses, supported by major scientific societies, drafted the first CTAS guidelines [77]. The following year, in 1999, the system was officially adopted and recommended nationally, thanks in part to the support of the Canadian Association of Emergency Physicians (CAEP) and the National Emergency Nurses Affiliation (NENA). A key innovation was the close collaboration between physicians and nurses, recognizing the crucial role of both in the triage process.

In subsequent years, CTAS showed a remarkable capacity to evolve. In addition to CAEP and NENA, further development was driven by the Association des médecins d'urgence du Québec (AMUQ); the Canadian Paediatric Society (CPS), which promoted the Paediatric CTAS in 2001; and the Society of Rural Physicians of Canada (SRPC), which ensured continuous attention to rural and remote settings [87].

This network of collaborations transformed CTAS into a national organizational model, capable of standardizing practice, reducing variability, improving safety, and providing a solid basis for research, training, and health system planning.

4.5.3   System Objectives

CTAS was conceived to make the triage process in Canadian EDs more equitable, consistent, and effective [77].

Its primary objective is to ensure that patients receive care according to clinical priority, not order of arrival, thereby reducing the risk that potentially serious conditions are overlooked in favor of less urgent cases [77]. To achieve this, CTAS adopts a common language and shared criteria, standardizing the assessment of acutely ill patients across the country and aiming to limit inter-observer variability.

The system also seeks to improve safety and patient flow efficiency by optimizing resource management and reducing inappropriate waiting times. The use of target physician-assessment times for each level makes it possible to monitor service performance and identify organizational bottlenecks.

In summary, CTAS objectives go well beyond simply ordering patients in the waiting room: the system is structured to generate measurable outcomes, such as shorter waiting times for critical patients, increased safety of care, better resource allocation, and ongoing monitoring of the efficiency of the entire emergency care system.

4.5.4   Clinical Functioning of the System

CTAS is a five-level system that orders patients according to clinical urgency rather than time of arrival. Each level is associated with a target time for physician assessment, making CTAS simultaneously a clinical tool (priority for the individual patient) and an organizational tool (performance metrics for the ED) [87].

Since its original implementation, the operational focus has been on "time to physician" and on verifying target achievement through "fractiles," that is, the proportion of patients seen within the recommended time frame. These concepts allow safety and flow to be monitored without turning time targets into rigid legal standards of care.

4.5.5 Acuity Levels

CTAS comprises five levels of acuity, defined according to the patient's clinical condition. Each level corresponds to a different priority for assessment, decreasing as urgency decreases:

CTAS 1—Resuscitation: Patients in critical condition with an immediate threat to life or vital organs. They require immediate treatment, concomitant with assessment.

CTAS 2—Emergent: Patients with serious or unstable conditions who should be seen within 15 minutes.

CTAS 3—Urgent: Patients at risk of deterioration or with significant pain who should be assessed within 30 minutes.

CTAS 4—Less Urgent: Patients with problems that do not carry an immediate risk of deterioration, to be seen within 60 minutes.

CTAS 5—Nonurgent: Minor or chronic conditions that can safely wait up to 120 minutes.

These time frames are safety and equity targets rather than "legal maximum waiting times." Recent revisions have reiterated that these limits must be interpreted within a performance-management framework (fractile targets) and in conjunction with rigorous, objective application of the assignment criteria.

4.5.6 Decision-Making Process: How the Acuity Level Is Assigned

Assignment of the CTAS level follows a logical sequence that combines clinical observation, categorization of the presenting complaint, and application of modifiers:

I. Immediate Observation/"Look Test": On arrival, the triage nurse performs a rapid visual assessment: posture, color, breathing, and level of consciousness. If there are signs of vital compromise (absent breathing, obvious shock, or coma), CTAS 1 is assigned immediately.

II. Identification of the Presenting Complaint: In the absence of immediate life-threatening compromise, the process begins from the main reason for attendance. Based on the primary symptom, the patient is mapped onto the standardized CEDIS list (e.g., chest pain, shortness of breath, headache, head injury, pediatric fever). The 2004 revision structurally linked CTAS and CEDIS to make assignments more objective and reproducible.

III. Collection of Clinical Data and Vital Signs: Blood pressure, heart rate, respiratory rate, oxygen saturation, temperature, and neurological status (GCS) are recorded, and pain intensity is quantified. These elements form the basis for first-order modifiers.

IV. Application of First-Order Modifiers: Marked abnormalities in vital signs (hypotension, extreme tachycardia, very low oxygen saturation, high fever in pediatrics), severe pain (>7/10), or significant mechanisms of injury automatically raise the acuity level.

V. Assessment of Second-Order Modifiers: When vital signs do not fully capture the level of risk, second-order modifiers are applied—for example, in psychiatric presentations (suicidal ideation, risk of violence, acute psychosis) or in particular clinical scenarios (tearing chest pain suggestive of aortic dissection). Even with normal vital signs, these conditions require higher acuity levels.

VI. Assignment of the Highest Applicable Level: Integrating presenting complaint and modifiers, the highest level indicated by the criteria present is assigned. The time of assignment is recorded, starting the clock for the target time to physician assessment.

VII. Dynamic Reassessment: CTAS triage is a dynamic process. Patients in the waiting area are periodically reassessed, and acuity is updated according to their clinical evolution. A patient initially classified as CTAS 3 for abdominal pain may become CTAS 2 if hypotension or signs of septic shock develop [77, 83].

The system is intentionally conservative: in case of doubt, the more urgent level should be chosen.

4.5.7   Development and Internal Validation

CTAS did not arise as a purely theoretical exercise or as a simple adaptation of a foreign model; rather, it is the result of a process that integrates clinical experimentation, field observation, and professional consensus.

The group started from the principle that a triage system must be clinically justifiable and empirically verifiable. Construction of CTAS was therefore grounded in real-world data, with the aim of linking common clinical presentations in the ED to observable outcomes: need for life-saving interventions, likelihood of hospital admission, ICU transfer, early mortality, and time to time-sensitive treatments [88, 89].

By analyzing observed outcomes, the group identified severity thresholds most strongly associated with high clinical risk. Each acuity level was therefore associated with a target time to physician assessment (0, 15, 30, 60, and 120 minutes), defined as operational targets on which equity and flow efficiency could be measured [77, 83].

To avoid a bureaucratic reading of these times, the concept of the fractile was introduced, the proportion of patients seen within the recommended time window. The focus thus moved from the individual case to the overall behavior of the system, creating a bridge between clinical quality and organizational quality.

From a conceptual standpoint, CTAS represents a synthesis between objective data and professional judgment: it does not seek to replace clinical expertise with a rigid algorithm but instead provides a shared framework to support decision-making [77, 83]. From the first versions, it was explicitly stated that the triage nurse may "upgrade" the acuity level in the presence of doubt or discrepancies between objective data and clinical impression.

The initial phase of internal validation focused on consistency between assigned level and immediate outcomes: rates of admission, ICU transfer, life-saving interventions, and waiting times [1, 2, 77, 83, 90]. Data from studies showed that the scale orders patients in proportion to their actual severity, with a clear risk gradient: CTAS 1–2 patients had substantially higher rates of admission and life-saving interventions than those in the lower levels [1, 2].

In summary, CTAS was born at the intersection of clinical epidemiology, professional experience, and health system management: realistic, measurable, and adaptable qualities that explain its robustness and longevity on the international stage.

4.5.8   External Validation After Implementation

Following its national adoption in 1999, CTAS underwent extensive empirical evaluation both in Canada and abroad. Attention focused on: Inter-observer reliability: agreement between different clinicians and clinical validity: the ability of CTAS levels to predict objective outcomes (mortality, critical illness, hospital admission, ICU admission, life-saving interventions) [1, 2, 82].

Regarding reliability, reported kappa values of 0.67, indicating substantial but not optimal agreement [82]. Only a few studies report values above 0.8, highlighting that inter-observer variability remains a critical issue, influenced by training, setting, and methodology [44].

Clinical validity appears overall more robust: for the ED mortality, more than 90% of patients who die in the ED are classified as CTAS 1–2 [1, 2].

Another element of construct validity is the association with admission and resource use: all studies show a monotonic gradient of increasing probability of admission and treatment intensity from Level 5 to Level 1. However, cases of under-triage are not negligible: a variable proportion of patients who were eventually admitted had initially been classified as CTAS 4–5 [1, 2, 91]. This phenomenon, which reflects differences in case mix, training, and local organization, underlines the importance of regular audits and targeted educational programs.

Overall, the literature confirms the robustness of CTAS and its distinctive feature: the combined use of presenting complaints and modifiers generates a risk gradient that is coherent with clinical outcomes and with realistic time targets, particularly in highly symptomatic cases. The system is not infallible, especially for conditions that are initially subtle, but its performance improves with periodic reassessment, careful attention to red flags, and structured programs of training [77, 83].

4.5.9   Role of the Triage Nurse

CTAS assumes that triage is performed by a specifically trained nurse. This is not incidental but a deliberate organizational and cultural choice [77, 83].

The nurse is the professional who first takes charge of the patient upon arrival in the emergency department: they gather initial information, observe obvious clinical signs, and formulate a rapid judgment on access priority.

Not all nurses can perform this role. CTAS triage requires specific training on the system, substantial experience in emergency and urgent care, advanced technical skills, rapid decision-making ability, strong communication skills with patients and families, and aptitude for managing emotionally and organizationally high-pressure situations.

The triage nurse must have an in-depth knowledge of CTAS and its tools: the CEDIS list, first- and second-order modifiers, and reassessment protocols [77, 83].

A crucial component is dynamic reassessment: monitoring patients in the waiting area, detecting early deterioration, and adjusting the assigned level. This demands constant vigilance and strong organizational skills.

At an organizational level, the distribution of patients across CTAS levels directly influences ED flow, activates specific care pathways, and can trigger diagnostic work-up even before physician assessment. Triage thus becomes both a clinical and managerial act, and the nurse who performs it is a key figure for the safety of individual patients and for the overall efficiency of the emergency care system.

4.5.10   Special Populations

CTAS recognizes that certain populations require a tailored assessment while maintaining the general five-level decision structure. For pediatric patients, a parallel system, Paediatric CTAS (PaedCTAS), has been developed and officially endorsed, produced jointly by CAEP and the Canadian Paediatric Society [92, 93]. The underlying logic remains identical, but thresholds and descriptors are adapted to age and pediatric physiology.

In gynecological and obstetric populations, CTAS retains the same priority structure but introduces dedicated modifiers for pregnancy-related conditions: vaginal bleeding, abdominal pain, reduced fetal movements, suspected pre-eclampsia, and others [77, 83]. These criteria, formalized in more recent revisions, are designed to avoid under-triage of potentially critical conditions such as first-trimester hemorrhage or early eclampsia. The decision-making approach remains the same but is enriched by special attention to maternal–fetal risk and the need for parallel care pathways.

4.5.11 Strengths and Clinical Advantages

CTAS has several key strengths: high degree of standardization, and it is a structured, sequential system that guides the triage nurse step by step, reducing errors due to subjective interpretation. Starting from a standardized presenting complaint, enriched by parametric modifiers, ensures that each patient is framed using a common language that is comparable across clinicians and settings.

4.5.11.1 Integration of Vital Signs and Pain

Incorporating vital signs and pain intensity into the decision process was a genuine innovation in the late 1990s and anticipated the modern use of Early Warning Scores [77, 83]. Urgency is determined not only by the symptom itself but also by its objectively quantifiable severity, making priority more closely aligned with actual risk.

It reports balance between standardization and clinical judgment; the system provides a shared framework but leaves room for "controlled subjectivization," whereby the nurse can upgrade priority in the presence of clinical factors not fully captured by recorded parameters. This balance makes CTAS flexible and suitable for complex presentations.

The system has periodic revisions that have integrated new clinical knowledge and updated criteria, keeping the system aligned with current evidence. This dynamic nature makes it ready for integration with digital tools, predictive scores, and, in the future, with artificial intelligence algorithms.

Taken together, CTAS offers a mature model that successfully combines scientific rigor, clinical usefulness, and organizational value.

4.5.12 Limitations and Clinical Drawbacks

Alongside its strengths, CTAS also presents several limitations. CTAS has an intrinsic complexity; the combination of presenting complaints with first- and second-order modifiers makes the system far from intuitive for those who are not adequately trained.

Second, not all nurses can apply it correctly; experienced professionals with advanced training are required, which limits its immediate applicability in less structured environments.

Another limitation is the residual interpretive variability, which, despite standardized criteria, judging the weight of vital sign abnormalities and interpreting second-order modifiers remains highly subjective. This contributes to non-negligible rates of over-triage and reduced specificity. The system tends to perform best in high-resource settings, where individual interpretation is naturally biased toward a cautious, inclusive approach.

CTAS requires time for application; the process requires complete measurement of vital signs, careful data collection, and evaluation of modifiers. In overcrowded emergency departments this can become a bottleneck, with a risk of delays in acuity assignment.

Finally, CTAS cannot be learned superficially; it requires courses, simulations, and periodic updates. Without solid and ongoing training, the risk of under- or overestimation of severity remains high.

4.5.12.1 Dependence on Available Resources

In small hospitals or rural settings with limited staff and heavy workloads, rigorous application of CTAS may be difficult. In such cases, the system risks becoming a largely formal exercise, with limited real impact on patient safety.

References

1. Hinson JS, Martinez DA, Cabral S, et al. Triage performance in emergency medicine: a systematic review. Ann Emerg Med. 2019;74(1):140–52. https://doi.org/10.1016/j.annemergmed.2018.09.022.
2. Zachariasse JM, van der Hagen V, Seiger N, Mackway-Jones K, van Veen M, Moll HA. Performance of triage systems in emergency care: a systematic review and meta-analysis. BMJ Open. 2019;9(5):e026471. Published 2019 May 28. https://doi.org/10.1136/bmjopen-2018-026471.
3. Kuriyama A, Urushidani S, Nakayama T. Five-level emergency triage systems: variation in assessment of validity. Emerg Med J. 2017;34(11):703–10. https://doi.org/10.1136/emermed-2016-206295.
4. Christ M, Grossmann F, Winter D, Bingisser R, Platz E. Modern triage in the emergency department. Dtsch Arztebl Int. 2010;107(50):892–8. https://doi.org/10.3238/arztebl.2010.0892.
5. Australasian College for Emergency Medicine. Guidelines on the implementation of the Australasian Triage Scale in emergency departments. Version 6 (G24). Australasian College for Emergency Medicine; 2023.
6. FitzGerald G, Jelinek GA, Scott D, Gerdtz MF. Emergency department triage revisited. Emerg Med J. 2010;27(2):86–92. https://doi.org/10.1136/emj.2009.077081.
7. Considine J, Ung L, Thomas S. Triage nurses' decisions using the National Triage Scale for Australian emergency departments. Accid Emerg Nurs. 2000;8(4):201–9. https://doi.org/10.1054/aaen.2000.0166.
8. Pardey TG. The clinical practice of emergency department triage: application of the Australasian triage scale—an extended literature review: part i: evolution of the ATS. Australas Emerg Nurs J. 2006;9(4):155–62. https://doi.org/10.1016/j.aenj.2006.09.003.
9. Considine J, LeVasseur SA, Charles A. Development of physiological discriminators for the Australasian Triage Scale. Accid Emerg Nurs. 2002;10(4):221–34. https://doi.org/10.1016/s0965-2302(02)00156-x.
10. Ebrahimi M, Heydari A, Mazlom R, Mirhaghi A. The reliability of the Australasian Triage Scale: a meta-analysis. World J Emerg Med. 2015;6(2):94–9. https://doi.org/10.5847/wjem.j.1920-8642.2015.02.002.
11. Dilley SJ, Standen P. Victorian nurses demonstrate concordance in the application of the National Triage Scale. Emerg Med. 1998;10(1):12–8. https://doi.org/10.1111/j.1442-2026.1998.tb00484.x.
12. Gerdtz MF, Chu M, Collins M, et al. Factors influencing consistency of triage using the Australasian Triage Scale: implications for guideline development. Emerg Med Australas. 2009;21(4):277–85. https://doi.org/10.1111/j.1742-6723.2009.01197.x.
13. Khanal B, Lewis O, Lewis M, Newbury J, Malla G. The Australasian Triage Scale applied in a tertiary care hospital in Nepal. Emerg Med Australas. 2005;17(1):88–9. https://doi.org/10.1111/j.1742-6723.2005.00680.x.

14. Chamberlain DJ, Willis E, Clark R, Brideson G. Identification of the severe sepsis patient at triage: a prospective analysis of the Australasian Triage Scale. Emerg Med J. 2015;32(9):690–7. https://doi.org/10.1136/emermed-2014-203937.

15. Visser LS, Montejano AS, Monetjano AS. Fast facts for the triage nurse: an orientation and care guide in a nutshell. New York: Springer Publishing Company; 2015.

16. Australian Commission on Safety and Quality in Health Care. Emergency triage education kit. 2nd ed. Sydney: Australian Commission on Safety and Quality in Health Care; 2024. Accessed 29 Dec 2025.

17. McCarthy M, McDonald S, Pollock W. Triage of pregnant women in the emergency department: evaluation of a triage decision aid. Emerg Med J. 2013;30(2):117–22. https://doi.org/10.1136/emermed-2011-200752.

18. Considine J, LeVasseur SA, Villanueva E. The Australasian Triage Scale: examining emergency department nurses' performance using computer and paper scenarios. Ann Emerg Med. 2004;44(5):516–23. https://doi.org/10.1016/j.annemergmed.2004.04.007.

19. Krey J. Klinische Ersteinschätzung in der Notaufnahme. Vergleichende evaluation 4 international bestehender Triagesysteme [triage in emergency departments. Comparative evaluation of 4 international triage systems]. Med Klin Intensivmed Notfmed. 2016;111(2):124–33. https://doi.org/10.1007/s00063-015-0069-0.

20. Twomey M, Wallis LA, Thompson ML, Myers JE. The South African Triage Scale (adult version) provides reliable acuity ratings. Int Emerg Nurs. 2012;20(3):142–50. https://doi.org/10.1016/j.ienj.2011.08.002.

21. Soogun S, Naidoo M, Naidoo K. An evaluation of the use of the South African Triage Scale in an urban district hospital in Durban, South Africa. S Afr Fam Pract. 2017;59(4):133–7. https://doi.org/10.1080/20786190.2017.1307908.

22. Bateman C. Answering when opportunity knocks - SATS goes global. S Afr Med J. 2012;102(3 Pt 1):121–2. Published 2012 Feb 23. https://doi.org/10.7196/samj.5534.

23. Dalwai M, Valles P, Twomey M, Nzomukunda Y, Jonjo P, Sasikumar M, et al. Is the South African Triage Scale valid for use in Afghanistan, Haiti and Sierra Leone? BMJ Glob Health. 2017;2:e000160. https://doi.org/10.1136/bmjgh-2016-000160.

24. Elbaih AH, Elhadary GK, Elbahrawy MR, Saleh SS. Assessment of the patients' outcomes after implementation of South African triage scale in emergency department, Egypt. Chin J Traumatol. 2022;25(2):95–101. https://doi.org/10.1016/j.cjtee.2021.10.004.

25. Twomey M, Cheema B, Buys H, et al. Vital signs for children at triage: a multicentre validation of the revised South African Triage Scale (SATS) for children. S Afr Med J. 2013;103(5):304–8. https://doi.org/10.7196/samj.6877.

26. Wangara AA, Hunold KM, Leeper S, et al. Implementation and performance of the South African Triage Scale at Kenyatta National Hospital in Nairobi, Kenya. Int J Emerg Med. 2019;12(1):5. Published 2019 Feb 11. https://doi.org/10.1186/s12245-019-0221-3.

27. Marombwa NR, Sawe HR, George U, et al. Performance characteristics of a local triage tool and internationally validated tools among under-fives presenting to an urban emergency department in Tanzania. BMC Pediatr. 2019;19(1):44. Published 2019 Feb 1. https://doi.org/10.1186/s12887-019-1417-7.

28. Rominski S, Bell SA, Oduro G, Ampong P, Oteng R, Donkor P. The implementation of the South African Triage Score (SATS) in an urban teaching hospital. Ghana Afr J Emerg Med. 2014;4(2):71–5. https://doi.org/10.1016/j.afjem.2013.11.001.

29. Wasingya-Kasereka L, Nabatanzi P, Nakitende I, et al. Two simple replacements for the triage early warning score to facilitate the South African Triage Scale in low resource settings. Afr J Emerg Med. 2021;11(1):53–9. https://doi.org/10.1016/j.afjem.2020.11.007.

30. Twomey M, de Sá A, Wallis LA, Myers JE. Inter-rater reliability of the South African Triage Scale: assessing two different cadres of health care workers in a real time environment. Afr J Emerg Med. 2011;1(3):113–8. https://doi.org/10.1016/j.afjem.2011.08.003.

31. Rosedale K, Smith ZA, Davies H, Wood D. The effectiveness of the South African Triage Score (SATS) in a rural emergency department. S Afr Med J. 2011;101(8):537–40. Published 2011 Jul 25.

32. Naidoo DK, Rangiah S, Naidoo SS. An evaluation of the triage early warning score in an urban accident and emergency department in KwaZulu-Natal. South Afr Fam Pract. 2014;56(1):69–73. https://doi.org/10.1080/20786204.2014.10844586.

33. Meyer GD, Meyer TN, Gaunt CB. Validity of the South African Triage Scale in a rural district hospital. Afr J Emerg Med. 2018;8(4):145–9. https://doi.org/10.1016/j.afjem.2018.07.004.

34. Goldstein LN, Morrow LM, Sallie TA, et al. The accuracy of nurse performance of the triage process in a tertiary hospital emergency department in Gauteng Province, South Africa. S Afr Med J. 2017;107(3):243–7. Published 2017 Feb 27. https://doi.org/10.7196/SAMJ.2017.v107i3.11118.

35. Mulindwa F, Blitz J. Perceptions of doctors and nurses at a Ugandan hospital regarding the introduction and use of the South African Triage Scale. Afr J Prim Health Care Fam Med. 2016;8(1):e1–7. Published 2016 Mar 29. https://doi.org/10.4102/phcfm.v8i1.1056.

36. Gyedu A, Agbedinu K, Dalwai M, et al. Triage capabilities of medical trainees in Ghana using the South African Triage Scale: an opportunity to improve emergency care. Pan Afr Med J. 2016;24:294. Published 2016 Aug 3. https://doi.org/10.11604/pamj.2016.24.294.8728.

37. McAlpine DJ, Hodkinson P, Fleming J. Pre-hospital over-triage and potential contributing factors in Cape Town, South Africa. S Afr J Pre-hospital Emerg Care. 2020;1(2):6–12.

38. Mullan PC, Torrey SB, Chandra A, Caruso N, Kestler A. Reduced overtriage and undertriage with a new triage system in an urban accident and emergency department in Botswana: a cohort study. Emerg Med J. 2014;31(5):356–60. https://doi.org/10.1136/emermed-2012-201900.

39. Gilboy N, Tanabe P, Travers D, Rosenau AM. Emergency severity index (ESI): a triage tool for emergency department care, version 4. In: Implementation handbook, vol. 2012; 2012. p. 12–0014.

40. Eitel DR, Travers DA, Rosenau AM, Gilboy N, Wuerz RC. The emergency severity index triage algorithm version 2 is reliable and valid. Acad Emerg Med. 2003;10(10):1070–80. https://doi.org/10.1111/j.1553-2712.2003.tb00577.x.

41. Tanabe P, Gimbel R, Yarnold PR, Kyriacou DN, Adams JG. Reliability and validity of scores on the emergency severity index version 3. Acad Emerg Med. 2004;11(1):59–65. https://doi.org/10.1197/j.aem.2003.06.013.

42. Emergency Nurses Association. Emergency severity index handbook: Fifth Edition (ESI v5). Schaumburg: Emergency Nurses Association; 2023. Accessed 29 Dec 2025. https://media.emscimprovement.center/documents/Emergency_Severity_Index_Handbook.pdf.

43. Mirhaghi A, Heydari A, Mazlom R, Hasanzadeh F. Reliability of the emergency severity index: meta-analysis. Sultan Qaboos Univ Med J. 2015;15(1):e71–7.

44. Worster A, Gilboy N, Fernandes CM, et al. Assessment of inter-observer reliability of two five-level triage and acuity scales: a randomized controlled trial. CJEM. 2004;6(4):240–5. https://doi.org/10.1017/s1481803500009192.

45. Travers DA, Waller AE, Katznelson J, Agans R. Reliability and validity of the emergency severity index for pediatric triage. Acad Emerg Med. 2009;16(9):843–9. https://doi.org/10.1111/j.1553-2712.2009.00494.x.

46. Lim BJV, Wahab SFA, Kueh YC. Validity and reliability of emergency severity index and conventional three-tier triage system in the emergency department, Hospital Universiti Sains Malaysia. Malays J Med Sci. 2020;27(2):90–100. https://doi.org/10.21315/mjms2020.27.2.10.

47. Storm-Versloot MN, Ubbink DT, Chin a Choi V, Luitse JS. Observer agreement of the Manchester Triage System and the emergency severity index: a simulation study. Emerg Med J. 2009;26(8):556–60. https://doi.org/10.1136/emj.2008.059378.

48. Chi CH, Huang CM. Comparison of the Emergency Severity Index (ESI) and the Taiwan triage system in predicting resource utilization. J Formos Med Assoc. 2006;105(8):617–25. https://doi.org/10.1016/S0929-6646(09)60160-1.

49. Green NA, Durani Y, Brecher D, DePiero A, Loiselle J, Attia M. Emergency severity index version 4: a valid and reliable tool in pediatric emergency department triage. Pediatr Emerg Care. 2012;28(8):753–7. https://doi.org/10.1097/PEC.0b013e3182621813.

50. Cairós-Ventura LM, de Las Mercedes Novo-Muñoz M, Rodríguez-Gómez JÁ, Ortega-Benítez ÁM, Ortega-Barreda EM, Aguirre-Jaime A. Validity and reliability of the emergency severity

index in a Spanish Hospital. Int J Environ Res Public Health. 2019;16(22):4567. Published 2019 Nov 18. https://doi.org/10.3390/ijerph16224567.

51. Grossmann FF, Nickel CH, Christ M, Schneider K, Spirig R, Bingisser R. Transporting clinical tools to new settings: cultural adaptation and validation of the emergency severity index in German. Ann Emerg Med. 2011;57(3):257–64. https://doi.org/10.1016/j.annemergmed.2010.07.021.

52. Tanabe P, Gilboy N, Travers DA. Emergency severity index version 4: clarifying common questions. J Emerg Nurs. 2007;33(2):182–5.

53. Platts-Mills TF, Travers D, Biese K, et al. Accuracy of the emergency severity index triage instrument for identifying elder emergency department patients receiving an immediate life-saving intervention. Acad Emerg Med. 2010;17(3):238–43. https://doi.org/10.1111/j.1553-2712.2010.00670.x.

54. Gilboy N, Tanabe P, Travers DA. The emergency severity index version 4: changes to ESI level 1 and pediatric fever criteria. J Emerg Nurs. 2005;31(4):357–62. https://doi.org/10.1016/j.jen.2005.05.011.

55. Sax DR, Warton EM, Kene MV, et al. Emergency severity index version 4 and triage of pediatric emergency department patients. JAMA Pediatr. 2024;178(10):1027–34. https://doi.org/10.1001/jamapediatrics.2024.2671.

56. Mackway-Jones K, Marsden J, Windle J, editors. Emergency triage: Manchester Triage Group. 3rd ed. Wiley; 2013.

57. Gräff I, Goldschmidt B, Glien P, et al. The German version of the Manchester triage system and its quality criteria--first assessment of validity and reliability. PLoS One. 2014;9(2):e88995. Published 2014 Feb 24. https://doi.org/10.1371/journal.pone.0088995.

58. Zaboli A, Sibilio S, Cipriano A, Park N, Bonora A, Pfeifer N, Giudiceandrea A, Brigo F, Turcato G. Italian validation of the Manchester Triage System towards short-term mortality: a prospective observational study. Emerg Care J. 2023;19(3):11443. https://doi.org/10.4081/ecj.2023.11443.

59. Olofsson P, Gellerstedt M, Carlström ED. Manchester Triage in Sweden - interrater reliability and accuracy. Int Emerg Nurs. 2009;17(3):143–8. https://doi.org/10.1016/j.ienj.2008.11.008.

60. Zaboli A, Sibilio S, Magnarelli G, et al. Daily triage audit can improve nurses' triage stratification: a pre-post study. J Adv Nurs. 2023;79(2):605–15. https://doi.org/10.1111/jan.15521.

61. Azeredo TR, Guedes HM, Rebelo de Almeida RA, Chianca TC, Martins JC. Efficacy of the Manchester Triage System: a systematic review. Int Emerg Nurs. 2015;23(2):47–52. https://doi.org/10.1016/j.ienj.2014.06.001.

62. Cicolo EA, Nishi FA, Peres HHC, Cruz DALMD. Effectiveness of the Manchester Triage System on time to treatment in the emergency department: a systematic review. JBI Evid Synth. 2020;18(1):56–73. https://doi.org/10.11124/JBISRIR-2017-003825.

63. Ausserhofer D, Zaboli A, Pfeifer N, Siller M, Turcato G. Performance of the Manchester Triage System in patients with dyspnoea: a retrospective observational study. Int Emerg Nurs. 2020;53:100931. https://doi.org/10.1016/j.ienj.2020.100931.

64. Parenti N, Reggiani ML, Iannone P, Percudani D, Dowding D. A systematic review on the validity and reliability of an emergency department triage scale, the Manchester Triage System. Int J Nurs Stud. 2014;51(7):1062–9. https://doi.org/10.1016/j.ijnurstu.2014.01.013.

65. van Veen M, Teunen-van der Walle VF, Steyerberg EW, et al. Repeatability of the Manchester Triage System for children. Emerg Med J. 2010;27(7):512–6. https://doi.org/10.1136/emj.2009.077750.

66. Grouse AI, Bishop RO, Bannon AM. The Manchester Triage System provides good reliability in an Australian emergency department. Emerg Med J. 2009;26(7):484–6. https://doi.org/10.1136/emj.2008.065508.

67. Mirhaghi A, Mazlom R, Heydari A, Ebrahimi M. The reliability of the Manchester triage system (MTS): a meta-analysis. J Evid Based Med. 2017;10(2):129–35. https://doi.org/10.1111/jebm.12231.

68. Souza CC, Chianca TCM, Cordeiro Júnior W, Rausch MDCP, Nascimento GFL. Reliability analysis of the Manchester Triage System: inter-observer and intra-observer agree-

ment. Rev Lat Am Enfermagem. 2018;26:e3005. Published 2018 Jul 16. https://doi.org/10.1590/1518-8345.2205.3005.

69. Gräff I, Latzel B, Glien P, Fimmers R, Dolscheid-Pommerich RC. Validity of the Manchester Triage System in emergency patients receiving life-saving intervention or acute medical treatment-a prospective observational study in the emergency department. J Eval Clin Pract. 2019;25(3):398–403. https://doi.org/10.1111/jep.13030.

70. Gräff I, Goldschmidt B, Glien P, Dolscheid-Pommerich RC, Fimmers R, Grigutsch D. Validity of the Manchester Triage System in patients with sepsis presenting at the ED: a first assessment. Emerg Med J. 2017;34(4):212–8. https://doi.org/10.1136/emermed-2015-205309.

71. Zachariasse JM, Kuiper JW, de Hoog M, Moll HA, van Veen M. Safety of the Manchester Triage System to detect critically ill children at the emergency department. J Pediatr. 2016;177:232–237.e1. https://doi.org/10.1016/j.jpeds.2016.06.068.

72. Zaboli A, Sibilio S, Massar M, et al. Enhancing triage accuracy: the influence of nursing education on risk prediction. Int Emerg Nurs. 2024;75:101486. https://doi.org/10.1016/j.ienj.2024.101486.

73. Zaboli A, Brigo F, Magnarelli G, et al. Reproducibility of the Manchester Triage System: a multicentre vignette study. Emerg Med J. 2025;42(6):403–10. Published 2025 May 22. https://doi.org/10.1136/emermed-2024-214213.

74. Zachariasse JM, Maconochie IK, Nijman RG, et al. Improving the prioritization of children at the emergency department: updating the Manchester Triage System using vital signs. PLoS One. 2021;16(2):e0246324. Published 2021 Feb 9. https://doi.org/10.1371/journal.pone.0246324.

75. Zachariasse JM, Espina PR, Borensztajn DM, et al. Improving triage for children with comorbidity using the ED-PEWS: an observational study. Arch Dis Child. 2022;107(3):229–33. https://doi.org/10.1136/archdischild-2021-322068.

76. Zaboli A, Battisti D, Ziller M, Turcato G, Camporesi S. Can patients' characteristics influence triage errors? A quasi-experimental study. Int Emerg Nurs. 2025;81:101647. https://doi.org/10.1016/j.ienj.2025.101647.

77. Beveridge R, Clarke B, Janes L, et al. Implementation guidelines for the Canadian Emergency Department Triage & Acuity Scale (CTAS). Version 16. Published December 16, 1998. Accessed 30 Dec 2025. https://ctas-phctas.ca/wp-content/uploads/2018/05/ctased16_98.pdf.

78. Funakoshi H, Shiga T, Homma Y, et al. Validation of the modified Japanese triage and acuity scale-based triage system emphasizing the physiologic variables or mechanism of injuries. Int J Emerg Med. 2016;9(1):1. https://doi.org/10.1186/s12245-015-0097-9.

79. Kalan L, Chahine RA, Lasfer C. The effectiveness and relevance of the Canadian triage system at times of overcrowding in the emergency department of a Private Tertiary Hospital: A United Arab Emirates (UAE) study. Cureus. 2024;16(1):e52921. Published 2024 Jan 25. https://doi.org/10.7759/cureus.52921.

80. Leeies M, Ffrench C, Strome T, Weldon E, Bullard M, Grierson R. Prehospital application of the Canadian Triage and Acuity Scale by emergency medical services. CJEM. 2017;19(1):26–31. https://doi.org/10.1017/cem.2016.345.

81. Smith DT, Snyder A, Hollen PJ, Anderson JG, Caterino JM. Analyzing the usability of the 5-level Canadian Triage and Acuity Scale by paramedics in the prehospital environment. J Emerg Nurs. 2015;41(6):489–95. https://doi.org/10.1016/j.jen.2015.03.006.

82. Mirhaghi A, Heydari A, Mazlom R, Ebrahimi M. The reliability of the Canadian Triage and Acuity Scale: meta-analysis. N Am J Med Sci. 2015;7(7):299–305. https://doi.org/10.4103/1947-2714.161243.

83. Bullard MJ, Musgrave E, Warren D, et al. Revisions to the Canadian Emergency Department Triage and Acuity Scale (CTAS) guidelines 2016. CJEM. 2017;19(S2):S18–27. https://doi.org/10.1017/cem.2017.365.

84. Grafstein E, Bullard MJ, Warren D, Unger B, CTAS National Working Group. Revision of the Canadian Emergency Department Information System (CEDIS) presenting complaint list version 1.1. CJEM. 2008;10(2):151–73. https://doi.org/10.1017/s1481803500009878.

85. Bullard MJ, Chan T, Brayman C, et al. Revisions to the Canadian Emergency Department Triage and Acuity Scale (CTAS) guidelines. CJEM. 2014;16(6):485–9.
86. Bullard MJ, Unger B, Spence J, Grafstein E, CTAS National Working Group. Revisions to the Canadian Emergency Department Triage and Acuity Scale (CTAS) adult guidelines. CJEM. 2008;10(2):136–51. https://doi.org/10.1017/s1481803500009854.
87. Bergeron S, Bailey B. Paediatric CTAS. Can J Emerg Med. 2002;4(1):4–5. Published online May 21, 2015. https://doi.org/10.1017/S1481803500005960.
88. Gravel J, Manzano S, Arsenault M. Validity of the Canadian Paediatric Triage and Acuity Scale in a tertiary care hospital. CJEM. 2009;11(1):23–8. https://doi.org/10.1017/s1481803500010885.
89. Gravel J, Fitzpatrick E, Gouin S, et al. Performance of the Canadian Triage and Acuity Scale for children: a multicenter database study. Ann Emerg Med. 2013;61(1):27–32.e3. https://doi.org/10.1016/j.annemergmed.2012.05.024.
90. Lee JY, Oh SH, Peck EH, et al. The validity of the Canadian Triage and Acuity Scale in predicting resource utilization and the need for immediate life-saving interventions in elderly emergency department patients. Scand J Trauma Resusc Emerg Med. 2011;19:68. Published 2011 Nov 3. https://doi.org/10.1186/1757-7241-19-68.
91. Bullard MJ, Melady D, Emond M, et al. Guidance when applying the Canadian Triage and Acuity Scale (CTAS) to the geriatric patient: executive summary. CJEM. 2017;19(S2):S28–37. https://doi.org/10.1017/cem.2017.363.
92. Warren DW, Jarvis A, LeBlanc L, et al. Revisions to the Canadian Triage and Acuity Scale paediatric guidelines (PaedCTAS). CJEM. 2008;10(3):224–43.
93. Bergeron S, Gouin S, Bailey B, Amre DK, Patel H. Agreement among pediatric health care professionals with the pediatric Canadian triage and acuity scale guidelines. Pediatr Emerg Care. 2004;20(8):514–8. https://doi.org/10.1097/01.pec.0000136067.07081.ae.

In modern emergency care, triage systems are far more than a technical tool for ordering a waiting room [1, 2]. They constitute the first clinical function, the entry point to every care pathway, and the threshold at which a patient's complexity is condensed into an initial decision that orients the entire subsequent diagnostic-therapeutic process [3, 4]. An error or imprecision in this first evaluative act can echo throughout the clinical trajectory, generating delays, inappropriate care, evolutionary risks, and organizational overload [3, 5, 6]. Consequently, analyzing methodological differences among international systems is not a mere comparative exercise but an attempt to understand the deeper logics that govern triage and shape everyday practice far more than might appear at first glance [7]. Grasping these differences is essential for anyone approaching triage [7, 8]. A professional familiar with only one system may unconsciously mistake particular methodological choices for universal principles [7–10]. This chapter offers a systematic analysis of the conceptual and structural divergences among the five principal triage systems worldwide: ATS, CTAS, ESI, MTS, and SATS. The aim is to delineate the internal logics of the systems, highlighting points of contact but, above all, the differences that characterize their philosophy and clinical practice.

5.1 The Methodological Roots of Triage Systems

Every triage system is born of a specific context and a particular organizational need. This aspect is often overlooked in comparative work, which tends to level profoundly different systems as if they were variations on one template. In reality, ATS, CTAS, ESI, MTS, and SATS share an apparently similar five-level structure, yet they arise from radically different visions of what it means to assess urgency [9, 10]. Their methodological divergences are not the result of casual or merely technical choices; they express precise clinical and cultural identities that have shaped how each country chose to confront the problem of priority in the emergency

A. Zaboli, G. Turcato, *Triage Systems: Essential Knowledge for Emergency
Nurses and Physicians*, https://doi.org/10.1007/978-3-032-20825-5_5

department [10]. These conceptual roots become the first discriminant: only by understanding the scenario in which a system was created can one grasp its internal logic, underlying philosophy, and interpretation of urgency itself.

The ATS arose in an environment where clinical experience and the nurse's professional autonomy play a central role [11]. This led to a scale that does not privilege rigid algorithms or tightly codified pathways, but rather the provider's ability to interpret the situation as a whole [11]. The result is a system that assigns great importance to the nurse's interpretation, the capacity to detect signs of criticality, and immediacy of assessment. Its internal methodology remains centered on clinical judgment that is not bound by an overly structured process but oriented by descriptive criteria that frame the decision [11]. This philosophy makes ATS a system dependent on the triage nurse's experience, who becomes chiefly responsible for decision safety [11].

Very different in design is the CTAS. CTAS was born of the need to standardize an extremely vast and varied health system, hospitals separated by hundreds of kilometers, significant distributional differences between urban and rural areas, and interpretive fragmentation that produced variability in waiting times and outcomes [12, 13]. Hence, the need to build a robust methodological structure capable of ensuring that the priority assigned in a large metropolitan hospital would be coherent with that in a small rural facility. CTAS therefore takes on a strongly standardizing dimension, seeking to replace interpretive diversity with a common language [12, 13]. The choice to work through coded presenting complaints, integrated with modifiers based on vital signs, pain, age, and risk factors, reflects the need to harness clinical judgment within a more regulated fabric that reduces variability without cancelling the triagist's sensitivity [12–14]. The internal logic of CTAS is thus that of a system that channels professional experience into a rich and coherent methodological framework.

The ESI carries a completely different philosophy. It emerged not so much as a response to clinical shortcomings as a tool of organizational management in a context of growing pressure on ED access [15, 16]. The founding idea is that priority should be defined not only by current clinical severity but also by predicted consumption of diagnostic-therapeutic resources in the minutes or hours ahead [15–17]. This represents a radical methodological shift, transforming triage into an act of managerial prediction as well. The system assumes that optimal resource distribution, coupled with early interception of critical patients, can yield clinical benefits even without a purely physiologic categorization of severity [15–17]. Its internal logic is that of a model aiming at efficiency and sustainability, seeking to marry clinical dimensions with flow optimization.

The MTS represents the response to the opposite necessity: to guarantee uniform decisions within a heterogeneous, universalistic context [18]. MTS stems from the awareness that interpretive variability can significantly limit safety and equity [18]. The solution adopted is a highly algorithmic framework based on symptom-driven flowcharts that guide the triage nurse along predefined decision pathways [18, 19]. Discriminators, ordered by seriousness, are the principal criteria that lead to level assignment, minimizing discretion [18, 19]. The MTS methodology does not arise from distrust of clinical judgment but from the need for uniformity and reproducibility, privileging decision consistency even at the cost of some rigidity in patient management [18, 19].

In the SATS, the principal challenge is scarcity of resources, high patient volume, and the need to identify critical conditions rapidly through objective parameters [20–22]. SATS introduces a parametric score as a structural element of decision-making and combines it with clinical discriminators to avoid underestimating severe conditions without overt physiologic derangement [20–22]. Its internal logic is that of a system that must function reproducibly even without highly trained staff, while still providing adequate protection for critical patients [20–22].

5.2   Internal Logics and Decision Architecture

If the methodological roots explain the systems' genesis, their decision architecture reveals each model's true identity [7, 10]. Differences do not stop at the five final categories, which are merely the surface of a much more complex structure, but concern how systems lead the operator through decision pathways, which elements they prioritize, how they integrate subjective and objective data, what role they assign to clinical reasoning, and how much space they leave for standardization.

ATS, consistent with its original philosophy, presents a minimally structured decision model [11, 23]. Assessment follows an intuitive sequence, observation, collection of essential information, identification of instability, but the process is not driven by a rigid algorithm. The triage nurse uses experience to read the situation globally, quickly identify criticality, and assign a level [11, 23]. The decision process is not apparently complex, yet it presupposes a considerable cognitive load. The absence of predefined pathways means the professional must continuously integrate clinical, behavioral, and contextual signals, sifting relevant from irrelevant within seconds [11, 23].

CTAS, by contrast, builds its decision architecture on a set of articulated steps. Identification of the presenting complaint activates a series of modifiers applied hierarchically [13, 24, 25]. Severe vital-sign derangements, severe pain, vulnerability, traumatic mechanisms, or critical clinical factors assume a modular role, adding and layering progressively to refine the final priority [13, 24, 25]. In this context, the triagist is called to navigate a tiered logic that reduces variability and guides decisions with objective criteria. CTAS does not merely recognize immediate severity; it attempts to anticipate the risk of deterioration, integrating concepts such as evolution and potential instability. The decision process becomes multidimensional, where an individual sign takes meaning only within the overall picture [13, 24, 25].

ESI's internal logic differs profoundly from all others. Decision-making unfolds in two broad phases: the first intercepts critical or potentially unstable patients; the second estimates the number of diagnostic or therapeutic resources the patient will likely require [16, 26]. This biphasic structure serves the model's objective, distinguishing severe cases from those that will demand high care intensity [16, 26]. ESI therefore requires the triage nurse to assess both severity and clinical pathway complexity, estimating diagnostic and treatment needs. The logic is predictive, designed to optimize flow management and reduce the risk that complex patients will be channeled into inappropriately rapid pathways [16, 26].

MTS presents the most formalized decision structure. The entire system relies on applying flowcharts corresponding to the patient's chief complaint. Each flowchart has discriminators ordered by severity, clear, unambiguous criteria for assigning a level [18, 19]. The architecture leaves little room for free interpretation because it is built to guarantee high reproducibility [18, 19]. This yields a linear, guided decision process in which the triage nurse applies the prescribed pathway. The system's strength lies in reducing inter-rater variability, though the same characteristic can be limiting in atypical cases or when symptomatology does not map neatly onto a single flowchart [18, 27].

SATS combines a quantitative decision model, based on standardized parametric assessment, with a qualitative layer of clinical discriminators [21, 22]. The physiologic score provides an objective measure of current severity, while discriminators prevent serious conditions with relatively preserved physiology from being missed [21, 22, 28]. The decision architecture is therefore hybrid: physiology compels a relatively standardized classification, while the clinical component integrates elements not immediately quantifiable [21, 22, 28]. This combination is designed for contexts where the triagist may lack advanced specialization or where massive volumes require a system that is extremely rapid, reproducible, and effective.

In summary, triage systems' internal logics differ markedly. ATS privileges immediate clinical judgment; CTAS develops a stratified, modular logic; ESI adopts a predictive, resource-based approach; MTS follows a binding algorithmic framework; and SATS embraces a structured physiologic model. It is within these architectures that the differences seen in daily practice and outcomes take root.

5.3   The Role of Vital Signs and Physiology

One of the most distinctive elements among triage systems is how vital signs are used, interpreted, and integrated into decision-making. Despite their apparent centrality in clinical assessment, physiology does not carry the same methodological weight everywhere [10, 29]. The place accorded to vital signs reveals each model's underlying philosophy and its conception of physiology's predictive value in determining clinical risk [10, 29].

In ATS, vital signs are important but not determinative. The scale does not rely on rigid thresholds; abnormal values are interpreted within the overall assessment [11, 30]. This choice expresses explicit trust in clinical judgment and the nurse's ability to contextualize information [11, 30, 31]. A patient with moderate tachycardia, for example, may be classified differently depending on global impression, history, and general presentation [11, 30, 31]. Physiology thus takes on an interpretive role, supporting the decision without automatically determining it [11, 30, 31].

CTAS, instead, uses vital signs as true modifiers of priority [13, 32, 33]. They are not merely an additional element; they play a central role in refining urgency. Marked tachycardia, hypotension, high fever, reduced oxygen saturation, or significant respiratory changes trigger an automatic upgrade [13, 32, 33]. This methodological choice treats vital signs as objective indicators of evolutionary risk, integrated systematically into decisions [13, 32, 33]. CTAS recognizes that, though variable and influenced by many factors, vital signs are crucial for anticipating deterioration.

ESI gives vital signs a more marginal role [16, 26]. They intervene mainly to discriminate between ESI 2 and ESI 3 when borderline data suggest potential compromise [16, 26]. This approach is coherent with the system's organizational nature: if the main objective is to anticipate the complexity of the diagnostic-therapeutic path rather than to grade clinical severity per se, vital signs become secondary, not irrelevant, but not the model's core [16, 26]. The risk is that patients with relevant physiologic derangement might be assigned a less urgent level if their condition does not appear immediately critical [16, 26].

In MTS, vital signs are expressed through numerical values embedded within the specific flowchart selected by the nurse [18, 34, 35]. This is consistent with the model's algorithmic logic, though relevant vitals can be bypassed if the operator chooses an entirely inappropriate flowchart for the presentation [18, 34, 35]. Vital signs thus play an indirect role, mediated by the discriminators themselves, an arrangement that allows adaptation across contexts but can create ambiguity when the operator errs at the start of the process [18, 34, 35].

Finally, SATS makes parametric status the primary basis of decision-making [36]. Vital signs generate an objective score whose sum automatically assigns priority [22, 36]. This meets a precise methodological need: in settings with heavy access pressure and limited highly trained staff, parameters provide sufficient objectivity for reliable classification [22, 28, 36]. Clinical discriminators, added as correctives, prevent underestimation of patients with severe conditions but relatively preserved physiology [22, 28, 36].

Comparing these approaches reveals significant differences. ATS treats parameters interpretively; CTAS uses them structurally to upgrade priority; ESI limits parametric evaluation to a narrow role; MTS incorporates it indirectly via flowchart discriminators; SATS places it at the center of decision-making.

5.4   Different Approaches to Clinical Risk, Safety, and Error Protection

Risk is another central dimension differentiating triage systems. Each model interprets safety differently, constructing specific mechanisms to reduce the probability of critical errors [1, 7]. The choice to privilege sensitivity or specificity profoundly influences patient distribution across priority levels and determines organizational consequences [1, 7].

ATS adopts a prudence-oriented approach to risk. The lack of rigid thresholds and the centrality of clinical judgment push the system toward a physiologic over-triage considered acceptable to protect patients [11, 37, 38]. The principle is that, in doubt, it is preferable to assign a higher category than to risk underestimation [11, 37, 38]. The Australian system relies on the triage nurse ability to catch early signs of deterioration and tends to provide broad protection against critical error, even at the cost of swelling intermediate or high categories [11, 37, 38]. While this safeguards clinical safety, in very crowded settings it can overload higher-priority areas.

CTAS manages risk through a more sophisticated, stratified logic. First- and second-order modifiers are designed to capture both immediate and potential risk [13, 25]. In CTAS, risk is not binary but a set of interacting factors [13, 25]. The approach is multilayered and rests on the idea that priority should reflect not only current severity but also a condition's potential evolution [13, 25]. CTAS is among the most sensitive in detecting latent risk, especially when physiology has not yet mirrored severity [13, 25]. Modifiers linked to mental health, mechanism of injury, or specific clinical signs reflect the intent to integrate dimensions not immediately measurable, making CTAS a high-protection model [13, 25].

ESI interprets risk in a different dimension. ESI level 1, dedicated to identifying truly critical patients, provides effective protection for time-dependent conditions [9, 16, 39]. Beyond absolute emergencies, however, the system focuses more on resource prediction than evolutionary risk [16, 39]. This implies lower protection than other models in conditions where severity is not expressed by instability or by high resource needs. The philosophy privileges flow efficiency over maximal sensitivity to all forms of clinical risk, without negating safety, but striking a different balance between accuracy and sustainability [9, 16, 39].

MTS employs an algorithmic risk strategy. Safety depends on the breadth and clarity of discriminators [18, 27, 40, 41]. This ensures good protection in typical presentations but can be less sensitive in atypical or complex cases that do not fit neatly into a single flowchart [18, 27, 41]. MTS tends toward a mixed profile, good sensitivity in highly specific symptom patterns, and some over-triage in intermediate categories [18, 40, 41]. The rigidity that underpins reproducibility can become a limitation when managing subtler risks.

SATS, finally, centers its risk approach on rapidly identifying conditions with high deterioration risk [20, 22]. Clinical discriminators function as correctives, integrating elements not captured by the score [20, 22, 42, 43]. Oriented to safety in complex contexts, the South African model privileges high sensitivity, accepting lower specificity as a methodological compromise [20, 22, 42, 43].

Thus, risk management differs profoundly: ATS valorizes interpretive prudence; CTAS integrates protection against potential risk through modifiers; ESI balances risk with efficiency; MTS adopts an algorithmic risk posture; and SATS concentrates protection on parametric condition. These differences shape the triage nurse experience and bear on clinical outcomes and organizational efficiency.

5.5   The Triage Nurse Role Across Systems

The triage nurse's role is one of the clearest areas where methodological differences emerge [23, 44]. Although the general task of assessing the patient, gathering essential information, and assigning a priority level is common to all models, each system conceives and distributes clinical responsibility differently [23, 44–46]. The triage nurse is not merely a procedural executor but a professional with varying degrees of autonomy, interpretive judgment, cognitive load, and decisional latitude [23, 45, 46].

Within ATS, the triage nurse is conceived as a professional with very high clinical autonomy [11, 30]. The system's low algorithmicity transfers a substantial interpretive responsibility to the operator [11, 30]. The lack of predefined pathways does not imply an absence of method; it places clinical meaning on expert observation [11, 30]. The triage nurse must integrate vitals, nonspecific signs, global impression, brief history, and behavioral presentation within seconds, making decisions that can determine outcomes [11, 30, 47]. This autonomy is both strength and vulnerability: valuing professional judgment enables rapid recognition of atypical conditions, while dependence on experience can expose the system to inter-observer variability if training is not uniform [11, 30, 46, 47].

CTAS assigns a different function, more balanced between structured application and clinical interpretation [12, 13]. It is designed to accompany the operator through a decision pathway without forcing them either to "invent" a decision or to follow a rule blindly, guiding assessment with a modular structure while leaving room for professional sensitivity [12, 13, 48]. Interpreting modifiers requires a high level of clinical understanding, as many refer to conditions that are not immediately apparent and therefore require discernment and the ability to recognize the potential for clinical deterioration [12, 13, 48]. In CTAS, responsibility lies in correctly identifying the presenting complaint, accurately assessing vital signs, and appropriately interpreting second-order modifiers. These three components require competence, conceptual depth, and the ability to integrate complex clinical information [12, 13, 48].

ESI assigns the triage nurse a unique role: the operator must foresee the complexity of the care pathway, not only clinical severity [16, 49, 50]. ESI requires dual competence, early recognition of the critical patient, and the ability to predict clinical-organizational resource use [16, 49, 51]. The nurse estimates the number of diagnostic or therapeutic resources, anticipating radiology, lab work, consultations, and treatments [16, 49–51]. This is a non-trivial cognitive load, because resource prediction is probabilistic, relying on clinical experience, knowledge of hospital pathways, and intuition about case complexity [49–51].

In MTS, the role shifts closer to that of an "expert applier" of an algorithm [6, 18]. The system is built to minimize variability and ensure interpretive uniformity through structured flowcharts and discriminators [18]. This does not reduce the triage nurse to passivity; they must choose the correct flowchart, interpret discriminators precisely, and apply the hierarchical logic that assigns the final level [6, 18, 27, 52]. However, the cognitive load differs from ATS, CTAS, or ESI: attention moves from a global patient assessment to correct algorithm navigation. The triage nurse needs a regulatory competence, the ability to adhere faithfully to method, while retaining enough flexibility to perform justified overrides when cases escape the algorithmic frame [6, 18, 27, 52]. The result is a professional figure tasked with fewer interpretive and more procedural decisions, yet still responsible for vigilant control to avoid pitfalls and rigidity [6, 27, 52].

SATS introduces yet another model. The triage nurse works where measurement of vital signs is not an accessory but the heart of the system [20, 22]. The operator's primary task is to record vitals accurately, assign the physiologic score, and recognize any clinical discriminators requiring an upgrade [20, 22]. The professional profile demanded by SATS is precise, systematic, and methodical, solid technical skills and the ability to integrate physiologic data with a lean but accurate clinical reading [20, 22, 53, 54]. Here the triage nurse becomes a "qualified measurer" of parametric status while retaining critical judgment to identify clinical conditions not immediately reflected in the score [20, 22, 53, 54]. SATS reduces discretion in assessing parametric stability but reintroduces it in recognizing conditions that the score may miss [20, 22, 53, 54].

In sum, differences in how systems conceive the triage nurse role are not operational details; they are direct projections of the underlying methodologies. In ATS, the triage nurse is the evaluative fulcrum and guardian of safety; in CTAS, a complex analyst navigating clinical and contextual variables; in ESI, a predictor of pathway complexity; in MTS, a rigorous interpreter of a structured algorithm; and in SATS, a clinical-physiologic operator integrating measurement and judgment. Each model assigns a different role, shaping cognitive load, required training, error modes, and even the nature of patient interaction [6, 7, 55]. Understanding these differences is to understand triage's depth: beyond numeric scales and color levels, real triage is an advanced cognitive act, differentiated and radically molded by the system that sustains it [6, 7, 55]. The triage nurses decisions thus express not only personal competence but also the entire methodological architecture of the model in use.

References

1. Christ M, Grossmann F, Winter D, Bingisser R, Platz E. Modern triage in the emergency department. Dtsch Arztebl Int. 2010;107(50):892–8. https://doi.org/10.3238/arztebl.2010.0892. Epub 2010 Dec 17
2. Robertson-Steel I. Evolution of triage systems. Emerg Med J. 2006;23(2):154–5. https://doi.org/10.1136/emj.2005.030270.
3. Cooper RJ. Emergency department triage: why we need a research agenda. Ann Emerg Med. 2004;44(5):524–6. https://doi.org/10.1016/j.annemergmed.2004.07.432.
4. Freeman M, Robinson S, Scholtes S. Gatekeeping under congestion: an empirical study of referral errors in the emergency department. INSEAD Working Paper No. 2020/09/TOM. SSRN Electron J [Internet]. 2020 [cited 2025 Dec 9]. Available from: https://ssrn.com/abstract=3036999. https://doi.org/10.2139/ssrn.3036999.
5. Hitchcock M, Gillespie B, Crilly J, Chaboyer W. Triage: an investigation of the process and potential vulnerabilities. J Adv Nurs. 2014;70(7):1532–41. https://doi.org/10.1111/jan.12304. Epub 2013 Dec 23

6. Ausserhofer D, Zaboli A, Pfeifer N, Solazzo P, Magnarelli G, Marsoner T, Siller M, Turcato G. Errors in nurse-led triage: an observational study. Int J Nurs Stud. 2021;113:103788. https://doi.org/10.1016/j.ijnurstu.2020.103788. Epub 2020 Oct 8

7. Zachariasse JM, van der Hagen V, Seiger N, Mackway-Jones K, van Veen M, Moll HA. Performance of triage systems in emergency care: a systematic review and meta-analysis. BMJ Open. 2019;9(5):e026471. https://doi.org/10.1136/bmjopen-2018-026471.

8. Zaboli A. Establishing a common ground: the future of triage systems. BMC Emerg Med. 2024;24(1):148. https://doi.org/10.1186/s12873-024-01070-2.

9. Hinson JS, Martinez DA, Cabral S, George K, Whalen M, Hansoti B, Levin S. Triage performance in emergency medicine: a systematic review. Ann Emerg Med. 2019;74(1):140–52. https://doi.org/10.1016/j.annemergmed.2018.09.022. Epub 2018 Nov 22

10. Farrohknia N, Castrén M, Ehrenberg A, Lind L, Oredsson S, Jonsson H, Asplund K, Göransson KE. Emergency department triage scales and their components: a systematic review of the scientific evidence. Scand J Trauma Resusc Emerg Med. 2011;19:42. https://doi.org/10.1186/1757-7241-19-42.

11. Australasian College for Emergency Medicine (ACEM). Guidelines on the implementation of the Australasian Triage Scale in emergency departments (V6 G24). Australian College of Emergency Medicine; 2023.

12. Beveridge R, Clarke B, Janes L, Savage N, Thompson J, Dodd G, Murray M, Jordan CN, Warren D, Vadeboncoeur A. Implementation guidelines for the Canadian emergency department Triage & Acuity Scale (CTAS). Canadian Association of Emergency Physicians; 1998. p. 1–32.

13. Bullard MJ, Musgrave E, Warren D, Unger B, Skeldon T, Grierson R, van der Linde E, Swain J. Revisions to the Canadian emergency department triage and acuity scale (CTAS) guidelines 2016. Can J Emerg Med. 2017;19(S2):S18–27.

14. Beveridge R, Ducharme J, Janes L, Beaulieu S, Walter S. Reliability of the Canadian emergency department triage and acuity scale: interrater agreement. Ann Emerg Med. 1999;34(2):155–9.

15. Wuerz RC, Milne LW, Eitel DR, Travers D, Gilboy N. Reliability and validity of a new five-level triage instrument. Acad Emerg Med. 2000;7(3):236–42.

16. Gilboy N, Tanabe P, Travers D, Rosenau AM. Emergency severity index (ESI): a triage tool for emergency department care, version 4. Implementation handbook, vol. 2012; 2012. p. 12–0014.

17. Shelton R. The emergency severity index 5-level triage system. Dimens Crit Care Nurs. 2009;28(1):9–12. https://doi.org/10.1097/01.DCC.0000325106.28851.89.

18. Mackway-Jones K, Marsden J, Windle J. Emergency triage: Manchester triage group. Wiley; 2013.

19. Amthauer C, Cunha ML. Manchester triage system: main flowcharts, discriminators and outcomes of a pediatric emergency care. Rev Lat Am Enfermagem. 2016;24:e2779. https://doi.org/10.1590/1518-8345.1078.2779.

20. Gottschalk SB, Wood D, DeVries S, Wallis LA, Bruijns S. The cape triage score: a new triage system South Africa. Proposal from the cape triage group. Emerg Med J. 2006;23(2):149–53.

21. Twomey M, Wallis LA, Thompson ML, Myers JE. The south African triage scale (adult version) provides reliable acuity ratings. Int Emerg Nurs. 2012;20(3):142–50.

22. Rominski S, Bell SA, Oduro G, Ampong P, Oteng R, Donkor P. The implementation of the south African triage score (SATS) in an urban teaching hospital, Ghana. Afr J Emerg Med. 2014;4(2):71–5.

23. Gerdtz MF, Bucknall TK. Why we do the things we do: applying clinical decision-making frameworks to triage practice. Accid Emerg Nurs. 1999;7(1):50–7.

24. Hall JN, McCarron J, Toarta C, McLeod SL, CTAS National Advisory Committee and NENA Triage Committee. Canadian emergency department triage and acuity scale (CTAS) guidelines 2025. Can J Emerg Med. 2025:1–4.

25. Murray M, Bullard M, Grafstein E. Revisions to the Canadian emergency department triage and acuity scale implementation guidelines. Can J Emerg Med. 2004;6(6):421–7.

26. Wolf L, Ceci K, McCallum D, Brecher D. Emergency severity index handbook, vol. 36. Emergency Nurses Association; 2023.
27. Van der Wulp I, Van Baar ME, Schrijvers AJ. Reliability and validity of the Manchester triage system in a general emergency department patient population in The Netherlands: results of a simulation study. Emerg Med J. 2008;25(7):431–4.
28. Mould-Millman CN. Assessing use of the South African triage scale in the Western Cape government emergency medical services system.
29. Ingielewicz A, Rychlik P, Sieminski M. Drinking from the holy grail-does a perfect triage system exist? And where to look for it? J Pers Med. 2024;14(6):590. https://doi.org/10.3390/jpm14060590.
30. Australian Commission on Safety and Quality in Health Care. Emergency triage education kit—Australasian triage scale—descriptors for categories [Internet]. Sydney: ACSQHC; 2024 [cited 2025 Dec 10]. Available from: https://www.safetyandquality.gov.au/sites/default/files/2024-04/emergency_triage_education_kit_-australasian_triage_scale-_descriptors_for_categories.pdf
31. Australasian College for Emergency Medicine; College of Emergency Nursing Australasia. Joint statement: vital signs [Internet]. Melbourne: ACEM; 2024 [cited 2025 Dec 10]. Available from: https://acem.org.au/getmedia/e3ed668d-7fcb-46f3-bf1a-132d026eff7d/S904_ACEM_CENA_Joint_Statement_Vital_Signs_FINAL
32. Canadian Triage and Acuity Scale (CTAS). Prehospital CTAS manual [Internet]. Ottawa: CTAS; 2014 [cited 2025 Dec 10]. Available from: https://ctas-phctas.ca/wp-content/uploads/2018/05/pre-ctas_manual_2014_v1.5.pdf
33. Canadian Association of Emergency Physicians. Emergency department triage: module 3 slides [Internet]. Ottawa: CAEP; 2013 [cited 2025 Dec 10]. Available from: https://caep.ca/wp-content/uploads/2017/06/module_3_slides_v2.5b_2013.pdf
34. Zachariasse JM, Maconochie IK, Nijman RG, Greber-Platzer S, Smit FJ, Nieboer D, van der Lei J, Alves CF, Moll HA. Improving the prioritization of children at the emergency department: updating the Manchester triage system using vital signs. PLoS One. 2021;16(2):e0246324. https://doi.org/10.1371/journal.pone.0246324.
35. Guedes HM, Souza CC, Pinto D Jr, Morais SS, Chianca TC. Evaluation of vital signs by the Manchester triage system: expert agreement. Rev Enferm UERJ. 2017;25:e7506.
36. Emergency Medicine Society of South Africa. South African Triage Scale (SATS) manual [Internet]. Cape Town: EMSSA; 2012 [cited 2025 Dec 10]. Available from: https://emssa.org.za/wp-content/uploads/2011/04/SATS-Manual-A5-LR-spreads.pdf
37. Considine J, Ung L, Thomas S. Triage nurses' decisions using the National Triage Scale for Australian emergency departments. Accid Emerg Nurs. 2000;8(4):201–9.
38. FitzGerald G, Jelinek GA, Scott D, Gerdtz MF. Emergency department triage revisited. Emerg Med J. 2010;27(2):86–92. https://doi.org/10.1136/emj.2009.077081.
39. Sax DR, Warton EM, Mark DG, Vinson DR, Kene MV, Ballard DW, Vitale TJ, McGaughey KR, Beardsley A, Pines JM, Reed ME; Kaiser Permanente CREST (Clinical Research on Emergency Services & Treatments) Network. Evaluation of the emergency severity index in US emergency departments for the rate of mistriage. JAMA Netw Open. 2023;6(3):e233404. https://doi.org/10.1001/jamanetworkopen.2023.3404. Erratum in: JAMA Netw Open. 2024;7(6):e2423536. https://doi.org/10.1001/jamanetworkopen.2024.23536.
40. Storm-Versloot MN, Ubbink DT, Chin a Choi V, Luitse JS. Observer agreement of the Manchester triage system and the emergency severity index: a simulation study. Emerg Med J. 2009 Aug;26(8):556–60. https://doi.org/10.1136/emj.2008.059378.
41. Zachariasse JM, Seiger N, Rood PP, Alves CF, Freitas P, Smit FJ, Roukema GR, Moll HA. Validity of the Manchester triage system in emergency care: a prospective observational study. PLoS One. 2017;12(2):e0170811. https://doi.org/10.1371/journal.pone.0170811.
42. Soogun S, Naidoo M, Naidoo K. An evaluation of the use of the South African Triage Scale in an urban district hospital in Durban, South Africa. S Afr Fam Pract. 2017;59(4):133–7.
43. Wallis LA, Gottschalk SB, Wood D, Bruijns S, De Vries S, Balfour C. The cape triage score-a triage system for South Africa. S Afr Med J. 2006;96(1):53–6.

44. Gerdtz MF, Bucknall TK. Triage nurses' clinical decision making. An observational study of urgency assessment. J Adv Nurs. 2001;35(4):550–61. https://doi.org/10.1046/j.1365-2648.2001.01871.x.

45. Cioffi J. Decision making by emergency nurses in triage assessments. Accid Emerg Nurs. 1998;6(4):184–91. https://doi.org/10.1016/s0965-2302(98)90077-7.

46. Burgess L, Kynoch K, Hines S. Implementing best practice into the emergency department triage process. Int J Evid Based Healthc. 2019;17(1):27–35. https://doi.org/10.1097/XEB.0000000000000144.

47. Gerdtz M, Bucknall T. Australian triage nurses' decision-making and scope of practice. Aust J Adv Nurs. 2000;18(1):24–33.

48. McLeod SL, Thompson C, Borgundvaag B, Thabane L, Ovens H, Scott S, Ahmed T, Grewal K, McCarron J, Filsinger B, Mittmann N, Worster A, Agoritsas T, Bullard M, Guyatt G. Consistency of triage scores by presenting complaint pre- and post-implementation of a real-time electronic triage decision support tool. J Am Coll Emerg Physicians Open. 2020;1(5):747–56. https://doi.org/10.1002/emp2.12062.

49. Eitel DR, Travers DA, Rosenau AM, Gilboy N, Wuerz RC. The emergency severity index triage algorithm version 2 is reliable and valid. Acad Emerg Med. 2003;10(10):1070–80. https://doi.org/10.1111/j.1553-2712.2003.tb00577.x.

50. French S, Gordon-Strachan G, Kerr K, Bisasor-McKenzie J, Innis L, Tanabe P. Implementing the emergency severity index triage system in Jamaican accident and emergency departments. J Emerg Nurs. 2019;45(2):124–31. https://doi.org/10.1016/j.jen.2018.11.010. Epub 2018 Dec 24

51. Shabrandi N, Bagheri-Saveh MI, Nouri B, Valiee S. Accuracy of nurses' performance in triage using the emergency severity index and its relationship with clinical outcome measures. Emerg Care J. 2022;18(4)

52. Franco B, Busin L, Chianca TC, Moraes VM, Pires AU, Lucena AD. Association between Manchester Triage System discriminators and nursing diagnoses. Revista gaucha de enfermagem. 2018;39:e2017–0131.

53. Augustyn JE. The South African Triage Scale: a tool for emergency nurses: emergency medicine. Prof Nurs Today. 2011;15(6):24–9.

54. Goldstein LN, Morrow LM, Sallie TA, Gathoo K, Alli K, Mothopeng TM, Samodien F. The accuracy of nurse performance of the triage process in a tertiary hospital emergency department in Gauteng Province, South Africa. S Afr Med J. 2017;107(3):243–7. https://doi.org/10.7196/SAMJ.2017.v107i3.11118.

55. Yuliandari KP. A literature review in triage decision making: supporting novice nurses in developing their expertise. Belitung Nurs J. 2019;5(1):9–15.

Triage System Performance

6

A direct and definitive head-to-head comparison of the performance of the triage systems currently in use—the ESI, the MTS, the CTAS, the SATS, and the ATS—is not yet available [1–3]. Although the literature has produced numerous analyses of the discriminatory ability and accuracy of each model, the data remain fragmented and often hard to compare [1–3]. The main difficulty lies in the practical impossibility, at least to date, of applying two or more systems simultaneously to the same cohort of real patients in a prospective, controlled fashion [1–3]. This lack of solid comparative studies is a significant methodological limitation that prevents a rigorous assessment of which system is most effective in terms of accuracy, predictive capacity, and inter-observer reliability [2, 4]. Most of what we know comes from indirect studies conducted in different contexts, with heterogeneous populations and variable reference standards [2–4]. The absence of universally recognized indicators to measure triage outcomes is an additional obstacle [5, 6]. In the absence of a gold standard, studies rely on surrogate measures, such as need for admission, ICU access, or in-hospital mortality, which, though useful, do not fully capture triage's overall impact on prognosis and clinical management [5–8]. Attempts to fill these gaps have used simulated scenarios, clinical vignettes, or hypothetical cases [9, 10]. These methods standardize comparisons but suffer from limited external validity: decision-making in simulated conditions does not reproduce the complexity of a real emergency department, with time pressure, organizational constraints, and interactions with patients and multidisciplinary teams [9, 10]. Systematic reviews and meta-analyses of internationally validated five-level systems have tried to summarize existing data, generally showing substantial equivalence in overall discriminatory capacity [1, 3, 11]. Mean sensitivity for identifying high-priority patients ranges from 60% to 90%, while specificity in low-urgency patients often exceeds 80% [1, 3, 11]. These values, however, conceal marked heterogeneity driven not only by intrinsic system differences but also by application context, staff training levels, and population characteristics.

A. Zaboli, G. Turcato, *Triage Systems: Essential Knowledge for Emergency Nurses and Physicians*, https://doi.org/10.1007/978-3-032-20825-5_6

6.1 Accuracy of Triage Systems

In principle, accuracy is the most direct measure of a triage system's reliability: it reflects how closely emergency-department decisions match the patients' true clinical severity. Operationally, it is expressed as the proportion correctly classified and by the balance between two opposing errors: under-triage, assigning too low a level to a truly severe patient, and over-triage, placing a non-critical patient in an unnecessarily high category [12]. Both have major implications: the former endangers patient safety; the latter overloads the system and consumes scarce resources [12].

Recent studies have examined accuracy in depth, showing that the most widely used international models, ESI, MTS, CTAS, SATS and ATS, have overall validity ranging from moderate to good, though with substantial variability by context and population [1, 3]. None of these systems can be considered universally superior: each performs better in some domains and worse in others. One systematic review reported overall accuracy of 59.6–72.5% for ESI, 49.0% for both MTS and CTAS, and 46.2–58.3% for ATS [13]. These results suggest that, while performance is generally acceptable, there is ample room for improvement and a need for further comparative studies to identify more balanced and effective models [1, 13].

ESI has stood out in several settings as one of the more accurate systems. Validation studies report overall accuracy between 59.6% and 72.5%, with some contexts and populations exceeding 80% [14–16]. Under-triage rates of 13–15% and over-triage of 20–25% outline a relatively balanced profile between safety and efficiency [14–16]. ESI has also shown excellent ability to predict hospital resource use, the endpoint it was designed for, thus displaying superior "operational accuracy" when the outcome is resource consumption rather than mortality [14–16]. Overall, studies and reviews converge in describing ESI as generally accurate, though not without limitations: performance is weaker in complex subgroups such as older adults, patients with nonspecific symptoms, or those with multiple comorbidities, warranting caution in generalization [17].

The MTS shows slightly lower accuracy than some competitors, reflecting a delicate balance between clinical safety and operational efficiency. Reported overall accuracy typically ranges from 65% to 75% [18]. The system favors protection of the critically ill, lowering under-triage (averaging 8–10%) at the cost of higher over-triage, which can reach 30–40% [19]. This enhances safety but reduces efficiency and contributes to ED crowding. MTS performance varies by presentation: it maintains higher sensitivity in time-critical conditions such as chest pain and dyspnea, but accuracy drops in less specific pictures such as abdominal pain or general symptoms [20–22]. In sum, MTS is generally safe, thanks to its tendency to overestimate severity, but it is not optimal for efficiency, with considerable room to improve handling of intermediate categories.

CTAS likely occupies a structural middle ground, with overall accuracy around 70% [23]. It curbs under-triage well, generally below 10%, but with variable over-triage ranging from 20% to 40% depending on context [24]. It is particularly accurate in critically ill patients, as highlighted in pediatric studies reporting optimal performance [25]. Conversely, in low-urgency cases CTAS tends to overestimate severity, which in some settings can worsen rather than relieve crowding [26]. This variability reflects the system's strong dependence on the outcome considered and the application context. When endpoints are severe events (mortality or ICU admission), CTAS remains solid and reliable; in less severe cases, it tends to shift patients upward in priority, reducing overall efficiency. CTAS is therefore best characterized as accurate and robust for high-acuity patients, with evident limits for minor urgencies where over-classification can strain sustainability.

ATS has shown the greatest difficulties in balancing under- and over-triage, with generally lower overall accuracy, about 45–60% [27, 28]. Studies indicate under-triage can reach very high levels, up to 30%, implying that as many as one in three truly critical patients could be assigned too low a priority [13]. This is especially concerning in time-dependent conditions, where even modest delays may significantly worsen outcomes. Over-triage rates, by contrast, are relatively contained (15–20%), reflecting higher specificity and a lower likelihood of placing stable patients in urgent categories [13]. This profile can limit resource misuse but at the potential expense of clinical safety. Overall, ATS appears less accurate than other five-level models, privileging specificity over sensitivity and showing the strongest tendency to under-triage.

SATS presents a distinctive accuracy profile, likely shaped by the resource-limited environments for which it was designed: a compromise between protecting the critical patient and maintaining system efficiency [29]. Validation studies report overall accuracy around 60–70%, lower than ESI, MTS, and CTAS but still acceptable [20, 29, 31]. Under-triage rates are generally contained ($\approx$10–15%), ensuring most severely ill patients are not lost in the flow [29–31]. In return, over-triage frequently exceeds 40%, meaning many non-urgent patients are classified as priority, substantially impacting workload and resource use [29–31]. SATS can thus be viewed as a highly protective system suited to patient safety in low-resource countries, with reduced operational accuracy in more structured systems where sustainability of flow is also paramount.

6.2 Discriminatory Capacity

Discriminatory capacity reflects how well a triage system separates high-priority from low-priority patients irrespective of total correct classifications. Methodologically, it is assessed via sensitivity, specificity, and the area under the ROC curve (AUROC) [32]. Sensitivity captures correct identification of critical cases; specificity captures correct identification of stable, non-urgent cases. AUROC offers an overall index of discrimination: values >0.70 are good, >0.80 very good, and near 1.0 excellent. An AUROC of 0.5 is equivalent to a coin toss [20–22, 32].

Overall, recent literature indicates that internationally validated five-level systems have, in general, good-to-very-good discriminatory capacity, with wide variation across contexts, populations, and clinical settings [1, 3]. A 2019 study showed sensitivity ranging between 60% and 90%, while specificity was generally above

80%. Differences between models remain substantial, and single-condition studies often polarize results in favor of one system or another [1, 3].

Across numerous validation studies, ESI displays a balanced discrimination profile, with a favorable mix of sensitivity and specificity. In major analyses, sensitivity clusters around 0.80–0.85 and specificity around 0.65–0.75, with AUROC commonly 0.75–0.80, placing ESI consistently among systems with good overall discrimination [1, 33]. Globally, sensitivity ranges from 60 to 90% and specificity often exceed 80%, confirming ESI's ability to detect most critical patients without excessive overestimation of stable ones [1]. ESI also performs best in predicting resource use, the outcome it was built for. In pediatrics, AUROC has approached 0.80 and outperformed ATS and MTS ($\approx$0.65–0.75), with particularly strong predictive capacity in critically ill children [1]. Performance is less robust in complex subgroups such as the elderly and those with atypical symptoms.

MTS shows slightly lower discriminatory capacity than ESI and favors safety at the expense of efficiency. Sensitivity generally ranges from 0.70 to 0.80, specificity 0.55–0.65, and AUROC averages 0.70–0.78, rarely exceeding 0.80 [1, 3]. Studies reveal wide variability: sensitivity 47–87% and specificity 84–94% depending on context and population, indicating strong dependence on organizational factors and application setting [1, 3]. MTS recognizes critical patients reasonably well but tends to misclassify a meaningful share of non-severe patients as urgent, reducing discriminatory efficiency, particularly in less specific conditions [34]. Conversely, in time-dependent diseases such as chest pain or dyspnea, sensitivity is high at the cost of lower specificity [20–22]. Performance is heterogeneous in vulnerable groups: pediatric precision may drop with nonspecific symptoms; in older adults, clinical complexity and comorbidity make high sensitivity harder to achieve. Results also vary with the chosen outcome (admission, mortality, diagnostic category), limiting generalizability. Overall, MTS is reliable for safety but less performant for discriminatory efficiency, especially in intermediate clinical conditions.

CTAS emerges as one of the strongest systems for discrimination. Numerous studies report AUROC between 0.72 and 0.76, with experiences exceeding 0.80, and sensitivity/specificity generally between 0.70 and 0.85 [1, 3]. This makes CTAS particularly reliable in correlating assigned levels with key outcomes such as hospital admission, ICU entry, and in-hospital mortality. Pediatric literature is especially favorable: pediatric CTAS has reached AUROC up to 0.96 for predicting ICU admission, indicating exceptional discrimination in critically ill children [35].

ATS shows the opposite profile: high specificity (often >80%), implying good identification of non-urgent patients, but lower sensitivity ($\approx$60–65%), with AUROC typically 0.65–0.70 [33, 36, 37]. This reflects the system's structure, anchored more to time targets than detailed clinical descriptors, favoring speed of application but reducing precision and amplifying subjective variability in ambiguous presentations [33, 36, 37].

SATS appears explicitly designed to maximize protection of the critically ill. Available data show sensitivity above 80% but lower specificity (<60%) and AUROC around 0.70, leading to systematic risk overestimation and over-triage above 40% [1, 29, 31]. This trade-off is considered acceptable in African systems, where the top priority is avoiding missed critical illness even at the expense of resource overuse [29, 31].

A recurrent cross-cutting finding is the influence of age on discrimination. In children, ESI and CTAS show higher AUROC (0.78–0.96) than ATS and MTS (0.65–0.67), indicating greater precision in recognizing pediatric critical illness [1, 3].

6.3   Inter-observer Reliability

Inter-observer reliability measures the extent to which different clinicians, faced with the same patient, reach the same urgency classification using the same system. It is crucial: even an accurate, discriminative system loses value if it cannot be applied uniformly. Agreement is typically quantified with Cohen's kappa (κ), where >0.6 denotes good agreement and >0.8 very good to excellent [38].

Evidence shows consistent differences among systems. CTAS emerges as one of the most reliable: several studies report κ between 0.70 and 0.80, averaging about 0.77 [39]. This "substantial" agreement likely reflects CTAS's structure, which combines objective symptom criteria with standardized physiologic parameters and detailed clinical descriptors, thereby reducing subjectivity and improving reproducibility.

ESI shows widely variable κ values (0.45–0.94), reflecting strong influences of context and training [10, 39, 40]. Centers with regular training and local calibration report excellent agreement (up to $\kappa = 0.94$) [10, 39, 40].

MTS typically yields κ between 0.61 and 0.70, with reports up to 0.95 in highly standardized settings [10, 18, 39]. Its complexity, though capable of flexibility, can amplify variability in borderline situations. Functioning nonetheless depends heavily on standardized implementation and regular training [9].

ATS shows lower reliability, with κ around 0.40–0.57, indicating only moderate agreement [19]. SATS shows even more variable reliability, with κ 0.55–0.70 [29, 30, 39].

Systematic reviews agree on two cross-cutting points. First, inter-observer reliability varies not only by system but also by population [1, 41]. Second, staff training is the key determinant of agreement [27]. Where programs of structured updates and simulation exist, κ values are consistently higher regardless of system. Reliability depends not only on a system's intrinsic properties but also on organizational context and training quality, a caution repeatedly emphasized in the literature.

6.4   Direct Comparison Studies

Head-to-head literature across five-level international systems is surprisingly scant and often methodologically fragile; few direct comparisons in the same populations allow robust performance evaluation.

In a single-center prospective study of 900 consecutively triaged patients with six trained nurses applying three systems in parallel and expert panel outcomes, under-triage was higher with ESI (86/421; 20%) than MTS (48/421; 11%) [42]. For all systems, sensitivity was low in the less urgent levels and specificity high in levels 1–2 (>92%) [42]. In another study, ESI showed more consistent performance than MTS, with AUROC in an acceptable range (0.68–0.84), while MTS results were more variable (0.60–0.97 with wide confidence intervals) [10]. For both systems, assigned urgency correlated with resource use, admission, and length of stay, supporting criterion validity; the two systems were judged comparably valid [10, 42].

A multicenter Dutch study compared MTS, ESI, and the national Dutch system in the same cohort of 696,518 visits (7 EDs in 6 hospitals) [43]. In the lowest-urgency level, ESI showed lower resource use, lower admission, and lower mortality than MTS, suggesting better ability to "keep low-risk patients low" [43]. The adjusted risk of admission rose more steeply with increasing urgency for ESI than MTS, indicating a sharper discriminatory gradient [43].

In a large metropolitan ED prospective parallel-group comparison of 12,000 adults, ESI was associated with significantly lower mortality, fewer complications, and fewer ICU admissions [44]. Patient satisfaction was also higher with ESI [44]. ESI's discrimination for key outcomes exceeded MTS. Under-triage was more frequent with ESI, while over-triage was higher with MTS [44]. ESI thus appeared to yield better overall clinical outcomes and efficiency at the cost of a slightly higher under-triage risk, whereas MTS was more protective of critical patients but less resource-efficient.

In a geriatric head-to-head comparison, MTS and ESI distributed urgency levels differently; level 3 classification was much more common with ESI (82.9%) than MTS (48.2%) [45]. Both systems are sensitive but imperfect in older adults, with under-triage risk in nonspecific presentations [45].

Overall, therefore, direct comparison studies across triage systems remain few, heterogeneous, and methodologically fragile; robust head-to-head designs are intrinsically difficult to implement because they require the simultaneous application of multiple scales to the same real-world patient population. As a consequence, current evidence allows only cautious, context-dependent inferences rather than definitive conclusions about the superiority of one system over another.

6.5 Comparisons Using Simulations and Vignettes

Comparisons based on clinical vignettes and simulated scenarios offer methodological rigor but an inevitably partial perspective. Synthetic cases standardize variables and ensure comparability across contexts and scales, reducing setting- and patient-specific noise. Yet this very artificiality introduces a structural bias: triage is stripped of uncertainty, time pressure, emotional load, and direct patient communication, elements integral to real practice. The risk is an idealized, "clean" portrait of system performance that is hard to overlay onto actual emergency departments.

Even so, available studies yield some comparative observations. SATS assessed with standardized vignettes showed mean sensitivity of 74% and specificity of 92%, with under-triage 14% and over-triage 12% [46]. MTS in European simulations showed "substantial" inter-observer reliability (κ 0.62) and high test-retest stability, but modest sensitivity (53.2%) for urgent cases and high under-triage in the elderly (25%) [47]. In a large MTS simulation, nurses' code-assignment error was 28.6%, with only moderate agreement with experts (κ 0.59) and lower predictive capacity versus "ideal" application [48]. Simulations of CTAS, ESI, and MTS showed good recognition of critical cases (levels 1–2) but poor accuracy in intermediate classes (levels 3–4), with substantial agreement limited to the highest urgencies [49]. Pediatric simulations showed MTS with higher sensitivity in children (83.3%) than in adults but still high under-triage. Comparative pediatric vignettes for ESI and CTAS reported similar performance: sensitivity 70–80% for critical conditions, specificity >90%, but notable difficulty correctly placing intermediate-severity children [50, 51].

Vignette-based work thus confirms that the major international systems reliably identify high-priority cases yet have important limitations in classifying intermediate urgencies, the category to which most ED patients belong. Simulations are valuable for controlled comparisons but cannot reproduce the complexity and pressures of real practice; results describe systems' theoretical potential rather than the concrete difficulties of crowded environments and variable clinical presentations.

6.6 Conclusions

Comparing the performance of ESI, MTS, CTAS, ATS, and SATS makes clear that none is universally superior across all clinical contexts. Each scale represents a compromise among accuracy, discriminatory capacity, and inter-observer reliability, calibrated to the health-system needs for which it was developed. Observed performance reflects not only intrinsic model characteristics but also clinical setting, geography and timing, and the operational aims that guided design.

ESI stands out for speed and impact on outcomes, with lower mortality and complications than MTS, albeit with slightly higher under-triage. MTS, conversely, offers more protection against under-triage at the price of high over-triage. CTAS is balanced, with good accuracy and high inter-observer reliability, though it tends to overestimate low-urgency cases. ATS privileges specificity over sensitivity, while SATS, born for low-resource contexts, maximizes sensitivity and accepts substantial over-triage.

The scientific literature, despite its breadth, has often approached triage with a degree of self-reference. Many studies focus on shoring up the validity of a national system, implicitly to support its diffusion, rather than conducting deep, cross-system comparisons. This limits the chance to highlight which features might be integrated to build a hybrid, more universal model. ESI's predictive power for resource use, MTS's safety in reducing under-triage, CTAS's inter-observer reliability, ATS's specificity, and SATS's sensitivity are all qualities that, if combined, could yield a more robust triage system adaptable to diverse contexts.

In short, current comparisons depict a heterogeneous landscape in which differences reflect health-system needs more than true methodological supremacy. Direct head-to-head studies remain too few; we need concurrent, same-patient comparisons to evaluate systems across the varied populations arriving in emergency departments. The future challenge is not to defend "one's own" model, but to pursue collaborative, comparative research capable of fusing the best features of existing systems to build tomorrow's triage: accurate, discriminative, reliable, and, above all, flexible across clinical and organizational realities.

References

1. Hinson JS, Martinez DA, Cabral S, George K, Whalen M, Hansoti B, Levin S. Triage performance in emergency medicine: a systematic review. Ann Emerg Med. 2019;74(1):140–52. https://doi.org/10.1016/j.annemergmed.2018.09.022. Epub 2018 Nov 22. PMID: 30470513.
2. Farrohknia N, Castrén M, Ehrenberg A, Lind L, Oredsson S, Jonsson H, Asplund K, Göransson KE. Emergency department triage scales and their components: a systematic review of the scientific evidence. Scand J Trauma Resusc Emerg Med. 2011;19:42. https://doi.org/10.1186/1757-7241-19-42. PMID: 21718476; PMCID: PMC3150303.
3. Zachariasse JM, van der Hagen V, Seiger N, Mackway-Jones K, van Veen M, Moll HA. Performance of triage systems in emergency care: a systematic review and meta-analysis. BMJ Open. 2019;9(5):e026471. https://doi.org/10.1136/bmjopen-2018-026471. PMID: 31142524; PMCID: PMC6549628.
4. Moll HA. Challenges in the validation of triage systems at emergency departments. J Clin Epidemiol. 2010;63(4):384–8. https://doi.org/10.1016/j.jclinepi.2009.07.009. Epub 2009 Oct 28. PMID: 19875271.
5. Zaboli A, Brigo F, Sibilio S, Brigiari G, Massar M, Parodi M, Mian M, Pfeifer N, Turcato G. What is the optimal outcome for evaluating the triage systems? Insights from a prospective observational study. Int Emerg Nurs. 2025;78:101540. https://doi.org/10.1016/j.ienj.2024.101540. Epub 2024 Nov 19. PMID: 39566440.
6. Zaboli A. Establishing a common ground: the future of triage systems. BMC Emerg Med. 2024;24(1):148. https://doi.org/10.1186/s12873-024-01070-2. PMID: 39148042; PMCID: PMC11328465.
7. Seiger N, Moll HA. Triage systems: outcome measures to validate. Ann Emerg Med. 2013;61(3):372–3. https://doi.org/10.1016/j.annemergmed.2012.09.013. PMID: 23433024.
8. Zachariasse JM, Nieboer D, Oostenbrink R, Moll HA, Steyerberg EW. Multiple performance measures are needed to evaluate triage systems in the emergency department. J Clin Epidemiol. 2018;94:27–34. https://doi.org/10.1016/j.jclinepi.2017.11.004. Epub 2017 Nov 14. PMID: 29154810.
9. Zaboli A, Brigo F, Magnarelli G, Gorick H, Garbin T, Clauser P, Sibilio S, Brigiari G, Massar M, Mian M, Pfeifer N, Turcato G. Reproducibility of the Manchester triage system: a multicentre vignette study. Emerg Med J. 2025;42(6):403–10. https://doi.org/10.1136/emermed-2024-214213. PMID: 40050005.
10. Storm-Versloot MN, Ubbink DT, Chin A, Choi V, Luitse JS. Observer agreement of the Manchester triage system and the emergency severity index: a simulation study. Emerg Med J. 2009;26(8):556–60. https://doi.org/10.1136/emj.2008.059378.
11. de Magalhães-Barbosa MC, Robaina JR, Prata-Barbosa A, Lopes CS. Validity of triage systems for paediatric emergency care: a systematic review. Emerg Med J. 2017;34(11):711–9. https://doi.org/10.1136/emermed-2016-206058. Epub 2017 Oct 4. PMID: 28978650.

12. Ausserhofer D, Zaboli A, Pfeifer N, Solazzo P, Magnarelli G, Marsoner T, Siller M, Turcato G. Errors in nurse-led triage: an observational study. Int J Nurs Stud. 2021;113:103788. https://doi.org/10.1016/j.ijnurstu.2020.103788. Epub 2020 Oct 8. PMID: 33120136.

13. Rasyid TA, Kosasih CE, Mirwanti R. The reliability and accuracy of international triage scale in the emergency department (ED): a literature review. J Nurs Care. 2020;3(1) https://doi.org/10.1186/s12245-015-0080-5.

14. Jordi K, Grossmann F, Gaddis GM, Cignacco E, Denhaerynck K, Schwendimann R, Nickel CH. Nurses' accuracy and self-perceived ability using the emergency severity index triage tool: a cross-sectional study in four Swiss hospitals. Scand J Trauma Resusc Emerg Med. 2015;23:62. https://doi.org/10.1186/s13049-015-0142-y. PMID: 26310569; PMCID: PMC4551516.

15. Mirhaghi A, Kooshiar H, Esmaeili H, Ebrahimi M. Outcomes for emergency severity index triage implementation in the emergency department. J Clin Diagn Res. 2015;9(4):OC04-7. https://doi.org/10.7860/JCDR/2015/11791.5737. Epub 2015 Apr 1. PMID: 26023578; PMCID: PMC4437092.

16. Shabrandi N, Bagheri-Saveh MI, Nouri B, Valiee S. Accuracy of nurses' performance in triage using the emergency severity index and its relationship with clinical outcome measures. Emerg Care J. 2022;18(4) https://doi.org/10.4081/ecj.2022.10638.

17. Grossmann FF, Zumbrunn T, Ciprian S, Stephan FP, Woy N, Bingisser R, Nickel CH. Undertriage in older emergency department patients–tilting against windmills? PLoS One. 2014;9(8):e106203. https://doi.org/10.1371/journal.pone.0106203. PMID: 25153120; PMCID: PMC4143318.

18. Parenti N, Reggiani ML, Iannone P, Percudani D, Dowding D. A systematic review on the validity and reliability of an emergency department triage scale, the Manchester Triage System. Int J Nurs Stud. 2014;51(7):1062–9. https://doi.org/10.1016/j.ijnurstu.2014.01.013. Epub 2014 Feb 2. PMID: 24613653.

19. Zachariasse JM, Seiger N, Rood PP, Alves CF, Freitas P, Smit FJ, Roukema GR, Moll HA. Validity of the Manchester triage system in emergency care: a prospective observational study. PLoS One. 2017;12(2):e0170811. https://doi.org/10.1371/journal.pone.0170811. PMID: 28151987; PMCID: PMC5289484.

20. Nishi FA, Polak C, Cruz DALMD. Sensitivity and specificity of the Manchester Triage System in risk prioritization of patients with acute myocardial infarction who present with chest pain. Eur J Cardiovasc Nurs. 2018;17(7):660–6. https://doi.org/10.1177/1474515118777402. Epub 2018 May 11. PMID: 29749756.

21. Ausserhofer D, Zaboli A, Pfeifer N, Siller M, Turcato G. Performance of the Manchester triage system in patients with dyspnoea: a retrospective observational study. Int Emerg Nurs. 2020;53:100931. https://doi.org/10.1016/j.ienj.2020.100931. Epub 2020 Oct 6. PMID: 33035878.

22. Zaboli A, Ausserhofer D, Pfeifer N, Magnarelli G, Ciccariello L, Siller M, Turcato G. Acute abdominal pain in triage: a retrospective observational study of the Manchester triage system's validity. J Clin Nurs. 2021;30(7–8):942–51. https://doi.org/10.1111/jocn.15635. Epub 2021 Jan 25. PMID: 33434346.

23. Rankin JA, Then KL, Atack L. Can emergency nurses' triage skills be improved by online learning? Results of an experiment. J Emerg Nurs. 2013;39(1):20–6. https://doi.org/10.1016/j.jen.2011.07.004.

24. Mirhaghi A, Heydari A, Mazlom R, Ebrahimi M. The reliability of the Canadian triage and acuity scale: meta-analysis. N Am J Med Sci. 2015;7(7):299–305. https://doi.org/10.4103/1947-2714.161243. PMID: 26258076; PMCID: PMC4525387.

25. Lee JY, Oh SH, Peck EH, Lee JM, Park KN, Kim SH, Youn CS. The validity of the Canadian triage and acuity scale in predicting resource utilization and the need for immediate life-saving interventions in elderly emergency department patients. Scand J Trauma Resusc Emerg Med. 2011;19:68. https://doi.org/10.1186/1757-7241-19-68. PMID: 22050641; PMCID: PMC3223131.

26. Gravel J, Fitzpatrick E, Gouin S, Millar K, Curtis S, Joubert G, Boutis K, Guimont C, Goldman RD, Dubrovsky AS, Porter R, Beer D, Doan Q, Osmond MH. Performance of the Canadian triage and acuity scale for children: a multicenter database study. Ann Emerg Med. 2013;61(1):27–32.e3. https://doi.org/10.1016/j.annemergmed.2012.05.024. Epub 2012 Jul 27. PMID: 22841173.
27. van der Wulp I. Reliability and validity of emergency department triage systems. Utrecht University; 2010.
28. Considine J, LeVasseur SA, Villanueva E. The Australasian triage scale: examining emergency department nurses' performance using computer and paper scenarios. Ann Emerg Med. 2004;44(5):516–23. https://doi.org/10.1016/j.annemergmed.2004.04.007. PMID: 15520712.
29. Twomey M, Wallis LA, Thompson ML, Myers JE. The south African triage scale (adult version) provides reliable acuity ratings. Int Emerg Nurs. 2012;20(3):142–50. https://doi.org/10.1016/j.ienj.2011.08.002. Epub 2011 Sep 17. PMID: 22726946.
30. Dalwai MK, Twomey M, Maikere J, Said S, Wakeel M, Jemmy JP, Valles P, Tayler-Smith K, Wallis L, Zachariah R. Reliability and accuracy of the south African triage scale when used by nurses in the emergency department of Timergara Hospital, Pakistan. S Afr Med J. 2014;104(5):372–5. https://doi.org/10.7196/samj.7604. PMID: 25212207.
31. Meyer GD, Meyer TN, Gaunt CB. Validity of the South African Triage Scale in a rural district hospital. Afr J Emerg Med. 2018;8(4):145–9. https://doi.org/10.1016/j.afjem.2018.07.004. Epub 2018 Jul 26. PMID: 30534518; PMCID: PMC6277536.
32. Hoo ZH, Candlish J, Teare D. What is an ROC curve? Emerg Med J. 2017;34(6):357–9. https://doi.org/10.1136/emermed-2017-206735. Epub 2017 Mar 16. PMID: 28302644.
33. van Veen M, Moll HA. Reliability and validity of triage systems in paediatric emergency care. Scand J Trauma Resusc Emerg Med. 2009;17:38. https://doi.org/10.1186/1757-7241-17-38. PMID: 19712467; PMCID: PMC2747834.
34. Azeredo TR, Guedes HM, Rebelo de Almeida RA, Chianca TC, Martins JC. Efficacy of the Manchester triage system: a systematic review. Int Emerg Nurs. 2015;23(2):47–52. https://doi.org/10.1016/j.ienj.2014.06.001. Epub 2014 Jun 18. PMID: 25087059.
35. Gravel J, Manzano S, Arsenault M. Validity of the Canadian Paediatric triage and acuity scale in a tertiary care hospital. CJEM. 2009;11(1):23–8. https://doi.org/10.1017/s1481803500010885. PMID: 19166636.
36. Chamberlain DJ, Willis E, Clark R, Brideson G. Identification of the severe sepsis patient at triage: a prospective analysis of the Australasian Triage Scale. Emerg Med J. 2015;32(9):690–7. https://doi.org/10.1136/emermed-2014-203937. Epub 2014 Dec 11. PMID: 25504659; PMCID: PMC4552895.
37. Forero R, Nugus P. Australasian College for Emergency Medicine (ACEM) literature review on the Australasian triage scale (ATS). Institute of Health Innovation; 2012.
38. van der Wulp I, van Baar ME, Schrijvers AJ. Reliability and validity of the Manchester Triage System in a general emergency department patient population in The Netherlands: results of a simulation study. Emerg Med J. 2008;25(7):431–4. https://doi.org/10.1136/emj.2007.055228. PMID: 18573959.
39. Pourasghar F, Tabrizi JS, Sarbakhsh P, Daemi A. Kappa agreement of emergency department triage scales; a systematic review and meta-analysis. J Clin Res Gov. 2014;3(2):124–33. https://doi.org/10.13183/JCRG.V3I2.78.
40. Grossmann FF, Nickel CH, Christ M, Schneider K, Spirig R, Bingisser R. Transporting clinical tools to new settings: cultural adaptation and validation of the Emergency Severity Index in German. Ann Emerg Med. 2011;57(3):257–64. https://doi.org/10.1016/j.annemergmed.2010.07.021. Epub 2010 Oct 16. PMID: 20952097.
41. Ingielewicz A, Szarafińska M, Grešner PM, Rychlik P, Zając M, Bielicki S, Stolarewicz T, Siemiński M. Comparative evaluation of the Manchester triage system and emergency severity index in predicting critical events in the emergency department. BMC Emerg Med. 2025; https://doi.org/10.1186/s12873-025-01420-8. Epub ahead of print. PMID: 41286624.
42. Storm-Versloot MN, Ubbink DT, Kappelhof J, Luitse JS. Comparison of an informally structured triage system, the emergency severity index, and the Manchester triage system to dis-

tinguish patient priority in the emergency department. Acad Emerg Med. 2011;18(8):822–9. https://doi.org/10.1111/j.1553-2712.2011.01122.x.

43. van Wegen ME, Fransen LFC, Thijssen WAMH, Alexandridis G, de Groot B. The association between urgency level and hospital admission, mortality and resource utilization in three emergency department triage systems: an observational multicenter study. Scand J Trauma Resusc Emerg Med. 2025;33(1):72. https://doi.org/10.1186/s13049-025-01392-5. PMID: 40312391; PMCID: PMC12044865.

44. Boğa E. The effects of patient triage management strategies on clinical outcomes and risk management in emergency departments: a prospective comparative study. Anatolian Curr Med J. 2025;7(1):8–14. https://doi.org/10.38053/acmj.1579702.

45. Ingielewicz A, Szarafińska M, Zając M, Brunka Z, Grażewicz M, Szczupak M, Siemiński M. Triage and hospitalization outcomes in the geriatric population of an emergency department: a retrospective cohort study comparing the Manchester triage system and the emergency severity index. PLoS One. 2025;20(9):e0332304. https://doi.org/10.1371/journal.pone.0332304. PMID: 40961061; PMCID: PMC12443246.

46. Twomey M, Wallis LA, Myers JE. Evaluating the construct of triage acuity against a set of reference vignettes developed via modified Delphi method. Emerg Med J. 2014;31(7):562–66. https://doi.org/10.1136/emermed-2013-202352.

47. van der Wulp I, van Baar ME, Schrijvers AJ. Reliability and validity of the Manchester Triage System in a general emergency department patient population in the Netherlands: results of a simulation study. Emerg Med J. 2008;25(7):431–34. https://doi.org/10.1136/emj.2007.055228.

48. Zaboli A, Brigo F, Magnarelli G, et al. Reproducibility of the Manchester Triage System: a multicentre vignette study. Emerg Med J. 2025;42(6):403–10. Published 2025 May 22. https://doi.org/10.1136/emermed-2024-214213.

49. Dippenaar E. Reliability and validity of three international triage systems within a private health-care group in the Middle East. Int Emerg Nurs. 2020;51:100870. https://doi.org/10.1016/j.ienj.2020.100870.

50. Bergeron S, Gouin S, Bailey B, Amre DK, Patel H. Agreement among pediatric health care professionals with the pediatric Canadian triage and acuity scale guidelines. Pediatr Emerg Care. 2004;20(8):514–18. https://doi.org/10.1097/01.pec.0000136067.07081.ae.

51. Travers DA, Waller AE, Katznelson J, Agans R. Reliability and validity of the emergency severity index for pediatric triage. Acad Emerg Med. 2009;16(9):843–49. https://doi.org/10.1111/j.1553-2712.2009.00494.x.

Part III

The Possible Future of Triage Systems

What Needs Improvement in Triage Systems

7.1 The Problem of "Good but Not Excellent" Discrimination

Triage systems are today one of the fundamental pillars of modern emergency department management [1, 2]. They represent the starting point of every clinical pathway and the critical decision threshold on which appropriate allocation of resources, patient safety, and, ultimately, the overall quality of care depend [2]. Effective triage not only regulates waiting times and the order of priority but directly influences clinical outcomes, patient satisfaction, and the organizational efficiency of the entire hospital system [2, 3].

Over the past three decades, five-level triage systems: the Canadian Triage and Acuity Scale (CTAS), the Australasian Triage Scale (ATS), the Emergency Severity Index (ESI), the Manchester Triage System (MTS), and the South African Triage Scale (SATS) have become universally recognized and validated tools, sharing a high degree of conceptual coherence [4–6]. All pursue the same objective: to provide a reliable classification of clinical severity within a very short time frame, ensuring uniformity and safety [4–6]. Despite their methodological differences, comparative analyses show a striking homogeneity in overall results: In terms of accuracy, reproducibility, and safety, the global performance of these systems is largely overlapping [4–6].

Behind this apparent convergence lies a common and persistent limitation, which can be described as the "0.7 paradox." Systematic reviews and validation studies published in recent years have consistently shown that, while maintaining good discriminatory ability, no triage system stably achieves values of area under the receiver operating characteristic curve (AUROC) above 0.8 [5, 6]. The discriminatory ability of a diagnostic or prognostic tool represents its capacity to distinguish correctly between subjects who do and do not have the condition of interest. In clinical practice, this characteristic is crucial, because it determines whether a test can accurately identify who is affected by a condition and who is not.

A. Zaboli, G. Turcato, *Triage Systems: Essential Knowledge for Emergency Nurses and Physicians*, https://doi.org/10.1007/978-3-032-20825-5_7

This capacity is usually summarized by statistical indicators such as sensitivity (true-positive rate), specificity (true-negative rate), and above all the AUROC, which provides an overall measure of discriminative performance across all possible decision thresholds [7, 8]. In practical terms, the AUROC expresses the probability that, when two subjects are chosen at random, one critically ill and one not, the system will assign a higher urgency level to the former. An AUROC of 0.5 corresponds to purely random discrimination, equivalent to a coin toss, while an AUROC of 1.0 represents perfect discrimination [8, 9].

Nearly all performance studies of triage systems show that overall discriminatory ability rarely exceeds an AUROC of 0.8. On the contrary, the literature quite consistently reports values below this threshold, indicating a global discriminative capacity that is "good" but not excellent [2, 4–6].

Despite the heterogeneity of geographical and organizational contexts, these figures outline a common picture: In real clinical practice, triage systems exhibit an average discriminative capacity that is "good" but systematically falls short of theoretical excellence [5, 6]. The threshold around 0.7–0.8 appears to constitute an empirical saturation point beyond which the models do not manage to progress, regardless of training, periodic revisions, or digital implementation. This raises an essential question: what prevents us from surpassing this limit? Is it a structural flaw of the systems themselves, a consequence of human variability, or an inevitable reflection of clinical complexity? If the algorithmic component of these tools is solid and validated, might the "missing 0.3" reside in the cognitive and contextual dimensions of triage, in the limitations of current evaluation metrics, or in the intrinsically probabilistic nature of clinical decision-making under uncertainty?

This needs to systematically analyze the determinants that may explain why triage systems fail to achieve excellent discriminative capacity. We therefore need to identify the internal and external components that contribute to this unrealized margin of performance and to explore realistic opportunities for intervention to address the "0.7 paradox." Understanding these factors is not merely of theoretical interest; it can offer concrete guidance for the development of corrective strategies and innovative models designed to improve the precision and reliability of triage systems while preserving their operational usability in complex, high-pressure environments [2].

Ultimately, it is possible that the "missing 0.3" does not represent an intrinsic defect of the models, but rather the inevitable reflection of the complex nature of emergency care, an arena in which human variability, clinical uncertainty, and rapidly evolving patient conditions make perfectly algorithmic discrimination impossible [10].

Awareness of this reality, however, should not diminish efforts toward improvement. On the contrary, it should act as a stimulus for ongoing scientific evolution and systematic updating of clinical practice.

7.1.1 Possible Causal Factors

The structural limit of triage systems, which consistently stabilizes around an AUROC of 0.7–0.8, cannot be interpreted as a simple technical failure or the consequence of a design error. Rather, it reflects the combined effect of multiple interconnected factors: organizational, cognitive, methodological, and clinical that converge at the very moment when the triage nurse must translate an often nebulous clinical picture into a rapid, binary decision [10, 11]. Understanding where the "missing 0.3" lies therefore requires exploration of the structural limits of the systems themselves, the complexity of human behavior and the intrinsic nature of emergency medicine.

7.1.2   Structural Problems

The first area of analysis concerns structural problems, that is, limitations inherent in the design and functioning of triage systems [5, 6]. These are critical issues that do not depend on the individual operator but on the model itself: its conceptual architecture and the decision logics on which it is based. It is within this dimension that many of the "systemic" causes of the 0.7 paradox are rooted [5, 10–12].

Basic architecture of the systems: One of the first elements to consider is the underlying philosophy with which triage systems were conceived. All models, CTAS, ESI, ATS, MTS and others, share a common ethical and methodological principle: Priority must be given to patient safety, even at the cost of overestimating severity [6, 10, 12, 13]. In other words, when in doubt, it is preferable to over-triage a patient than to underestimate their condition.

This approach has an unquestionable clinical and ethical value, but it carries a measurable side effect: a systematic increase in over-triage. Several studies report that over-triage rates in five-level systems fluctuate between 25% and 45% [5, 14–16]. This excess sensitivity, while safeguarding safety, reduces overall specificity and therefore the global discriminative capacity of the system. It is a delicate balance: The more the model shifts toward protection, the more its statistical precision is eroded.

Background noise: A second structural limitation concerns the management of non-specific presentations [17]. In an attempt to accommodate the full spectrum of clinical conditions, every triage system includes categories such as "non-specific" or "other." A very large proportion of patients is channeled into these labels: individuals without a clear leading symptom who may in fact have anything from mild, self-limiting problems to time-critical emergencies such as sepsis or pulmonary embolism [17–20]. These heterogeneous categories generate internal "diagnostic noise" that dilutes the discriminative power of the systems. As long as the algorithm cannot distinguish more finely within these groups, the ability to separate truly critical patients from physiologically stable, non-critical ones will remain intrinsically limited. It is likely that an important component of the "missing 0.3" lies exactly here: in the grey zone of atypical or multi-symptom presentations that escape the rigid logic of decision flowcharts [17–20].

Focus on the critical condition: A further structural limitation derives from the fact that triage systems are designed primarily to detect critical illness, not to measure the full spectrum of clinical severity with precision. Their primary objective is the prompt identification of life-threatening or time-dependent emergencies, operating under the implicit assumption that symptomatic severity corresponds to pathological severity [5, 6, 10, 12]. In reality, this equivalence is only partial. Many alarming presentations (such as intense pain or subjectively severe dyspnea) may, after diagnostic work-up, prove unrelated to life-threatening disease, whereas some serious conditions begin with minimal or atypical signs [5, 6, 10, 12]. As a consequence, triage systems tend to privilege sensitivity over specificity: They perform well in recognizing overt threats but lose discriminative capacity in borderline areas [5, 6].

A further paradoxical effect must be considered. When triage functions effectively and enables early treatment, the patient may not go on to develop a severe outcome, which then appears retrospectively, as measured by conventional metrics, as a "false positive" [10, 12]. In other words, successful prevention of adverse events can worsen the apparent statistical performance of the system.

Reference outcome: A further, often underestimated structural issue concerns the choice of the reference outcome used to measure the discriminatory capacity of triage [2, 10, 12]. The AUROC of a system depends directly on the type of endpoint selected as the "gold standard": The same model may show high values when tested against an outcome consistent with its underlying logic (e.g., resource utilization), but much lower values when evaluated against different indicators such as mortality or hospital admission [2, 10, 12]. It has been shown that, for the same patient cohort, changing the outcome can modify the AUROC by as much as 0.1–0.2 points, generating divergent interpretations of the very same performance [2, 5, 6, 10, 12]. This means that triage discrimination is not an absolute property, but a relational measure between the system and the outcome chosen. Evaluating a model designed to recognize clinical urgency against a delayed or multifactorial endpoint will inevitably weaken its statistical coherence. The definition of the reference outcome therefore represents a crucial element and is probably one of the key interpretative factors of the "0.7 paradox." This issue will be explored in a dedicated section, as it constitutes the most direct point of contact between system structure, evaluation metrics, and the clinical meaning of discrimination.

7.1.3 Human Factors

Alongside structural limitations, a substantial component of the "0.7 paradox" is linked to the human dimension of triage, that is, to the interaction between the professional and the system. No algorithm, however refined, operates autonomously [21–23]. The assignment of an acuity code always depends on the clinician's interpretation, on their perceptions, on the emotional context, and on the operational conditions in which the decision is made [21–23]. It is at this interface between rule and judgment that a significant proportion of the observed variability is generated.

Cognitive biases and decisional pressure: Triage decisions are made under conditions of extreme time and cognitive pressure. The clinician must evaluate, within a few minutes, information that is often incomplete, under stress, and in chaotic environments [23]. Under these circumstances, cognitive biases inevitably emerge, such as anchoring to first impressions, the tendency to overestimate recent or memorable conditions (availability heuristic), or framing effects, in which risk perception varies according to how the problem is presented [23, 24]. In addition, a defensive stance, "better to overestimate than to miss a critical case," may amplify over-triage [25]. These mechanisms are not individual faults but adaptive strategies of the brain under load; nevertheless, they reduce the overall consistency of the system.

Operational context and decision fatigue: Environmental conditions play an equally decisive role [23, 24]. Overcrowding, staff shortages, and the simultaneous management of multiple patients diminish the quality of attention and increase the likelihood of approximate or erroneous decisions. So-called decision fatigue, the cognitive exhaustion resulting from a high number of repeated choices, may lead either to automatized responses or, conversely, to excessive caution [23, 24, 26]. The timing of the shift also matters: The probability of error increases during night hours and periods of peak operational pressure, when available cognitive resources are dramatically reduced [21, 23].

7.1.4   Pathological Factors

The third interpretative axis of the "0.7 paradox" is represented by the biological and clinical variability of patients, a dimension that by its nature escapes the rigid codification of triage systems. Even a perfectly applied model cannot nullify the unpredictability with which disease manifests and evolves. It is within this patho-physiological complexity that an irreducible component of the discriminatory limit is rooted.

Atypical presentations and low-specificity syndromes: Many time-dependent conditions, such as sepsis, pulmonary embolism, or aortic dissection, initially present in a subtle, non-specific, or masked manner. In these early phases, vital signs may be normal and symptoms only weakly characteristic, inevitably leading to assignment of an intermediate priority. Conversely, conditions that are not life-threatening but symptomatically striking, such as, panic attacks, renal colic, acute vertigo, generate high scores because of subjective intensity rather than true vital risk. This asymmetry between symptom and severity is one of the main sources of systemic error: Triage interprets the clinical surface, not the underlying trajectory.

Frailty, comorbidity, and altered compensatory mechanisms: In older, frail, or multi-morbid patients, the clinical picture tends to be less noisy but more unstable [21, 27]. Sepsis without fever, myocardial infarction without pain, or respiratory failure masked by the bradykinesia typical of advanced age make the initial assessment particularly misleading. Reduced compensatory mechanisms and poor symptom expressiveness lead to underestimation of severity. In the opposite direction, patients with anxiety, chronic pain or functional disorders amplify the subjective perception of symptoms, contributing to frequent overestimation. These polarities attenuate the linearity of the relationship between clinical presentation and actual outcome, limiting the statistical precision of the system.

7.2   Outcomes for Evaluating Triage

Triage is the crucial point of entry in the care pathway of the acutely ill patient, a decision node that decisively shapes not only immediate clinical management but the entire care trajectory and, in many cases, the patient's final outcome [2]. Because of this centrality, triage systems, and even more so each single triage decision made by a professional, require rigorous, systematic, and comparable evaluation capable of measuring effectiveness, reliability, and impact on clinical outcomes for both the patient and the department [5, 6]. Yet triage evaluation remains a complex and debated field, lacking a universally shared language. Differences in the systems employed, in healthcare settings, in target populations, and in stated objectives make it difficult to define common, comparable outcome indicators [2]. The result is that, despite a broad and growing literature, we still lack a homogeneous and universally recognized metric to determine how "correctly" a triage has been performed and what the real impact of the assigned category is on a patient's clinical course [2, 5, 6].

Evaluating triage requires appropriate measurement tools that can explore, in an integrated way, two complementary dimensions. The first concerns the performance of the triage system as a whole: the ability of the algorithm and organizational structure to classify patients according to their true clinical urgency and to ensure a care flow consistent with established priorities [10, 12, 28]. The second, no less important, concerns the decision-making competence of the triage nurse: the correctness and clinical coherence of the assessment made at that precise moment, based on available information and the operational context [29–31]. Both dimensions need solid, valid, and shared outcomes able to answer the question every emergency system should ask: "Was this triage right or wrong?"

Answering that question is anything but simple. The "correctness" of triage is not an absolute value but a multidimensional construct that depends on clinical, temporal, and contextual variables. A triage may be appropriate from the standpoint of clinical priority yet inappropriate from a resource-management perspective, or vice versa. Moreover, the relationship between triage and the patient's final outcome is mediated by multiple factors: subsequent treatments, waiting times, resource availability, diagnostic errors, and even patient characteristics.

For example, in a patient presenting with chest pain or dyspnea, 30-day mortality might reasonably be used to judge whether the initial triage correctly recognized severity or whether under-triage delayed treatment [32]. The same indicator loses meaning for minor or self-limiting conditions where death is neither plausible nor attributable to the triage decision [10, 28]. Even in potentially serious conditions, 30-day mortality can be only partly attributed to triage, because the clinical course is influenced by many subsequent factors (pharmacologic treatment, procedures, inpatient care, comorbidities) [10]. Hence, a key methodological challenge in evaluating triage systems is identifying the "best outcome" on which to base judgments about triage effectiveness, remembering that any single triage result reflects both the intrinsic capacity of the system to function and the operator's ability to make it function. Research has proposed many outcomes, mortality, admission, resource use, waiting time, safety, and quality indicators, but there is still no international consensus on their hierarchy and interpretation [2, 28]. Harmonizing outcomes is not merely academic: It is a prerequisite for scientifically comparing systems, conducting reliable meta-analyses, and, above all, improving triage quality in daily practice. Only through shared, comparable indicators can we build a common language of triage that transcends national and institutional boundaries and translates the decision complexity of emergency care into performance metrics that are transparent, reproducible, and focused on patient safety.

Evaluating a triage system's effectiveness is one of the most complex methodological challenges in modern emergency medicine. Authors since the 2000s have argued that a good system should identify, early, patients who require time-critical treatment while avoiding unnecessary medicalization or urgent resource allocation to low-risk patients [2, 10–12]. Subsequent debate has emphasized that objective definitions of "benefit" and "harm" remain problematic, because there is no universally accepted gold standard for clinical urgency [2, 10–12]. This absence has pushed the literature toward multiple surrogate outcomes, validation endpoints that indirectly reflect a system's ability to discriminate urgency correctly.

Within this context, contributions by Kuriyama et al., and Challen mark key methodological steps [10, 12]. They clarified how triage "validation" can be conceived and measured, introducing two reference paradigms: criterion validity and construct validity. Criterion validity assumes that triage can be compared with an external standard of truth, such as an expert panel judgment or a predefined urgency/ severity classification, thus relying on comparison with an authority or formal codification. The intrinsic limit is clear: Expert judgment and predefined classifications are themselves subjective interpretations and may not rest on objective or reproducible parameters [2, 10, 12, 28]. One risks validating one subjective system with another, producing tautological rather than empirical validation.

Construct validity, by contrast, seeks to anchor triage evaluation to clinical or managerial outcome indicators with greater objectivity and measurability. Here, the quality of triage is inferred from its behavior against observable variables such as mortality, hospital admission, ICU admission, resource use, or waiting times. If the system is valid, there should be a proportional and coherent gradient between assigned priority and the severity of observed outcomes: Patients classified as more urgent should, on average, show higher rates of severe events or resource use. Even so, these "objective" clinical outcomes, mortality or ICU admission, do not fully capture the intrinsic complexity of urgency. Death or critical-care admission are extreme endpoints that may not reflect the initial severity at triage: A patient can survive thanks to timely treatment despite being initially at risk of death; conversely, the absence of a fatal outcome does not mean the initial state was "not severe" [10, 12]. It therefore becomes necessary to identify reliable surrogates for clinical severity that more sensitively and realistically represent the patient's risk at the time of assessment. As in other fields where what is measured is not fully objectifiable (e.g., pain assessment or psychiatric diagnosis), it may be possible in triage to construct standardized indicators that, though originating in subjective perception, become objective through consensus and reproducibility.

7.2.1 Main Outcomes for Evaluating Triage

Clinical outcomes are the most natural starting point, because they directly reflect the relationship between assigned priority and true clinical severity. At the same time, no single clinical endpoint can fully capture the complexity of "urgency." There remain, however, definitive and objective endpoints that often mark the extreme spectrum of acute severity.

1. Mortality: ED mortality, in-hospital mortality, or 28/30-day mortality are the most commonly used indicators in validation and comparative studies and are often used to judge individual triage decisions [5, 6, 28]. The strengths are their "hard," objective nature, and ease of ascertainment, which allow comparison across systems and verification of a coherent urgency gradient, mortality rising with higher assigned priority. The limits are substantial: Mortality is influenced by many factors that follow triage (therapeutic decisions, resource availability, comorbidities, patient attributes), which may over- or underestimate triage's true impact on survival [10]. It is also ill-suited to minor conditions, and short- to mid-term mortality (e.g., 30 days) may not be causally linked to the presenting complaint.

2. Hospital admission: Admission is the most frequently analyzed endpoint in the international literature [2, 5, 6, 28]. Its strengths lie in its generally coherent increase with higher triage priority, reflecting perceived severity and the need for further care; it is easy to record and enables direct comparisons among systems (ESI, CTAS, MTS) [5, 33, 34]. Its limits are the strong influence of hospital policies, bed capacity, and local admission practices, which reduce validity as a "pure" urgency indicator; it also fails to distinguish clinical necessity from precautionary or social admissions and is modulated by patient context.

3. ICU admission: ICU entry is a sensitive, specific outcome for acute severity and for the potential benefit of time-critical care; it is often used in high-income settings and may refine interpretation where intensity-of-care thresholds are salient [28]. Strengths include its close linkage to clinical severity and timeliness of care. Limits include wide variation in ICU thresholds across countries, hospitals, and even units, plus the fact that some critically ill patients receive intensive or step-up care outside formal ICUs. Contemporary practice has also made ICU use more selective, often later in hospitalization, so only a small fraction of acutely ill patients enters ICU [35]; many severe conditions are now managed effectively outside, reducing sensitivity as a direct measure of initial severity and limiting its

use as a sole validation outcome [35]. Do-not-intubate and other therapeutic-limitation populations also depress observed ICU and critical-event rates [35].

4. Critical events in the ED: These include cardiac arrest, intubation, shock, resuscitation, or rapid transfer to critical care [28, 36, 37]. They directly indicate the system's ability to recognize truly urgent, time-dependent states. They are, however, relatively rare, limiting their utility for large-scale evaluation or routine audit; their incidence is influenced by operational context, team response times, and protocol maturity.

5. Life-Saving Interventions (LSI) and Acute Medical Treatments: LSIs are immediate, time-dependent actions to prevent death or rapid deterioration (e.g., intubation, defibrillation, epinephrine or vasopressors, thrombolysis, urgent transfusion) [28, 38]. Acute Medical Treatments are urgent but not necessarily life-saving (e.g., IV analgesia, fluids, antibiotics, bronchodilators) delivered to stabilize or rapidly improve acute conditions [28, 38]. Their strengths are their proximity to the core notion of urgency and their ability to measure, directly and immediately, whether triage identified a need for urgent intervention. Recent authors propose these as more proximal and sensitive surrogates than mortality or simple admission [38]. The limits are the lack of uniform definitions across studies, settings, and organizational cultures. In some contexts, even low-complexity maneuvers are counted as LSIs, whereas in universalist, well-resourced systems, they are routine and thus weakly discriminative. The heterogeneity reflects resources, protocols, and team skill and raises a methodological issue: A one-size-fits-all LSI basket across syndromes (chest pain, dyspnea, syncope, trauma) may be too coarse, with loss of sensitivity (and sometimes specificity) [28]. Patient factors (frailty, comorbidities) also modulate observed LSI rates regardless of initial severity. In short, LSIs are more faithful to clinical urgency than ICU admission or generic "critical events," but they require shared standards (by setting and syndrome), case-mix adjustment, and a clear taxonomy distinguishing truly life-saving interventions from urgent but non-vital treatments.

Triage is not only about clinical priority; it is also an organizational tool to optimize flow, improve operational efficiency, and ensure equitable access [2]. Managerial/process outcomes reflect the impact of triage on the entire ED system rather than on individual patients, gauging how effectively limited resources are managed amid variable and rising demand. They can serve as indirect surrogates of triage quality; a well-functioning triage tends to reduce waits, hasten care for the most urgent, and improve departmental organization, yet focusing solely on managerial variables risks a partial picture: Efficiency is not synonymous with clinical quality or safety.

1. Waiting time: The interval between triage and first medical evaluation should show an inverse gradient with assigned priority [39]. Its strengths are intuitive meaning and ease of measurement; its limits are strong dependence on crowding, staffing, bed availability, and operational pressure, so it must be interpreted in context [39].

2. Time-to-treatment: The interval from triage category to the start of the indicated therapy or diagnostic-therapeutic action is closer to triage's clinical impact and bridges organizational and clinical outcomes [40]. It is pragmatic and meaningful, and shorter times for high-priority codes are often associated with better outcomes and fewer adverse events [40]. Measuring it is complex, heavily context-dependent, and shorter times do not automatically mean better quality (especially when over-triage is prevalent). Many conditions lack a universally agreed "correct timing"; classic STEMI metrics exist, but NSTEMI timing remains heterogeneous and protocol-driven [41, 42].

3. ED length of stay (LOS): LOS, from triage to discharge/admission, summarizes the whole process and signals system fluidity, disposition efficiency, and congestion [43]. It is influenced by many variables extrinsic to triage (inpatient bed availability, diagnostic turnaround, boarding) and should be read as a systemic indicator rather than a direct measure of triage validity [43–45].

4. Resource utilization: The number and type of tests, consultations, procedures, and nursing interventions per triage level reflect triage's impact on consumption and sustainability [46, 47]. Still, utilization is highly heterogeneous and sensitive to local practice patterns, policies, and technology; it does not separate appropriate from inappropriate use and does not linearly map to clinical urgency [46–48]. High resource use may mirror complexity rather than medical urgency. It is therefore a useful complementary lens on efficiency and usage patterns, but insufficient to define triage quality or correctness.

5. Left Without Being Seen (LWBS): The share of patients leaving before medical evaluation is an indirect but sensitive marker of perceived efficiency and congestion [49, 50]. It provides insight into crowding, reception quality, and whether lower-urgency patients are being managed in ways that discourage abandonment [49, 50]. It is influenced by many non-triage factors (waits, environment, communication, perceived severity), and a low LWBS does not necessarily indicate good triage; it may reflect over-prioritization, low volumes, or abundant resources [49, 50]. Severe cases rarely leave, so LWBS is largely decoupled from clinical urgency.

Going forward, triage evaluation should shift from purely descriptive/organizational measures to clinical-operational metrics that capture the real capacity, of both system and operator, to identify time-dependent diseases and evolution-risk conditions requiring timely care. The starting point is recognizing that triage is not merely for ordering flow; it is a clinical act that effectively sets a patient's "time-to-safety." Correct triage is the one that swiftly and accurately flags conditions where delay translates into concrete risk of deterioration, disability, or death—the heart of "urgency," that is, the time–prognosis relationship. Beyond classic time-critical conditions (STEMI, stroke, sepsis, major trauma, anaphylaxis), there is a wide area of time-sensitive disease where prompt diagnosis or treatment reduces suffering, complications, and illness duration (severe pain, asthma exacerbations, acute abdomens, early infections). The concept of urgency should therefore be broadened physiopathologically, not only prognostically.

Within this vision, judging whether triage was "right" or "wrong" cannot ignore the final diagnosis. Such judgment makes sense only once the underlying condition and its true temporal need are known. In other words, triage quality can only be fully understood ex post, when diagnosis is established and the patient's temporal requirement can be estimated [51]. One possibility can be that, at the end of the clinical course (including any admission), the responsible physician record a retrospective urgency corresponding to the level of timeliness that, in hindsight, would have been appropriate for that condition (e.g., "no urgency," "moderate urgency," "high urgency," or "time-critical") and indicate whether a clinically significant delay in care or treatment occurred relative to actual needs [28, 51]. Applied systematically, this would enable a system based on proximal, syndrome-specific outcomes rather than late endpoints like mortality or admission. The goal is to define indicators that are truly sensitive to clinical urgency, for example, delivery of a syndrome-specific acute treatment within a predefined window, or "time-to-key-action": the time from triage to the decisive intervention for that syndrome (antibiotics in sepsis, IV analgesia in severe pain, bronchodilator in asthma, coronary angiography in high-risk ACS). Standardized by disease and context, such indicators could be the new frontier of triage evaluation. Any such model must adjust for case-mix, frailty, comorbidities, and therapeutic limitations, and it must be sensitive to contextual factors (resources, crowding, and local protocols) that affect response times and access. Only with these adjustments can we ensure equitable evaluation and comparability across centers, avoiding penalties for systems operating under tougher conditions or with fewer resources. Ultimately, the future of triage evaluation should integrate clinic, time, and proximal outcomes so that the question "was this triage right or wrong?" is answered not by mortality or admission, but by the ability to recognize the real disease in time and anticipate its therapeutic need. One proposal can be related to recording retrospective urgency, and building syndrome-specific clinical–temporal indicators, this could be a first step toward progressive, pathology-by-pathology standardization that translates triage complexity into a shared, reproducible, and clinically meaningful metric.

7.3   Areas for Improvement in Triage Systems: Toward a Collaborative, Evidence-Based Approach

The contemporary scientific literature on triage reveals a significant epistemological paradox: Despite ongoing efforts to develop new prioritization systems, empirical evidence consistently shows that the five main validated systems (ATS, CTAS, ESI, MTS, and SATS) achieve broadly equivalent performance in terms of clinical outcomes, predictive accuracy, and patient safety [5, 6].

This phenomenon, documented in recent systematic reviews, suggests that the prevailing strategy of continually "reinventing" triage systems may be fundamentally ineffective and could represent a misuse of scientific and clinical resources. The systematic reviews conducted by Zachariasse et al. [6] and Hinson et al. [5], which together analyzed more than 200 studies published over the last two decades, showed that no newly proposed system has demonstrated clinically meaningful superiority over the existing validated frameworks [5, 6].

Taken together, these findings raise fundamental questions about current research and development strategies in the field of triage and point to the need for a paradigm shift: moving away from a model of fragmented innovation toward a collaborative, systematic improvement of the existing triage frameworks.

Over the past 15 years, the scientific literature has documented the continual development and proposal of new triage systems, each presented as an improvement over pre-existing models. However, critical appraisal of the available evidence shows that these systems do not demonstrate performance superior to their predecessors [2, 6]. The evolution of the five validated triage systems has been excessively fragmented, with each framework developing in relative isolation, drawing on context-specific evidence without any transversal integration of accumulated knowledge.

This sectorial approach, marked by a strong element of scientific "parochialism," has failed to generate meaningful progress in the overall landscape of triage systems, which remains substantially limited in its interpretive and predictive capacity. Such stagnation is attributable, to a large extent, to the absence of interdisciplinary and international teams engaging in structured, methodologically rigorous collaboration on the development and refinement of triage systems [2].

In contrast to other areas of emergency medicine, the field of triage is characterized by a lack of international scientific coordination. At present, there are no collaborative initiatives comparable to those led by major scientific societies for the development of shared European or international guidelines. This gap results in the absence of a common trajectory and a unified strategic vision for the evolution of triage systems.

It is therefore essential to promote international collaboration through the establishment of multidisciplinary, multinational teams dedicated to the systematic improvement of existing triage systems.

The current fragmentation gives rise to substantial cross-cutting problems. The language of triage is not uniform: Professionals in neighboring countries do not share the same methodological framework and, above all, lack adequate tools to engage in meaningful comparison on what should be a cornerstone of emergency medicine [31, 52].

To appreciate the magnitude of this issue, it is helpful to draw a parallel with other time-critical conditions. Imagine the management of a patient with STEMI or sepsis, in which each institution applied completely different treatment protocols despite sharing a common clinical definition. In a similar way, contemporary triage systems, although demonstrating broadly comparable performance, operate according to entirely different frameworks, thereby preventing the comparability of results and hindering the implementation of improvements based on transferable evidence.

The improvement of triage systems could be markedly accelerated through joint efforts and structured international comparison, following the model already established in other areas of emergency medicine.

Only through a paradigm shift that prioritizes collaboration over competition, and incremental refinement over fragmented radical innovation, will it be possible to achieve substantial progress in the ability of triage systems to ensure accurate, safe, and efficient prioritization of patients in the Emergency Department.

7.4   Triage Nurse Education: Current Gaps and Future Directions

The triage literature reveals a striking paradox: Although hundreds of studies have examined the performance and validation of triage systems, research on the ongoing education of triage nurses remains surprisingly scarce and fragmented. This imbalance represents a critical gap in the evidence base, because the accuracy of any triage system is intrinsically dependent on the competence of the professionals who apply it.

Inter-rater variability in triage, typically measured using Cohen's kappa, commonly ranges between 0.52 and 0.78 even within the same triage system, suggesting that operator-related factors contribute substantially to inconsistency in decision-making [5]. Yet the relationship between education, clinical experience, and performance remains poorly understood and is characterized by often contradictory findings in the existing literature [5, 53, 54].

At present, educational models for triage nurses vary markedly between jurisdictions, institutions, and even within a single health system [53, 54]. This heterogeneity is evident both in initial training and in continuing education.

With regard to initial training, course duration ranges from a few hours to multi-day programs. In some settings, training is limited to 4 h of mainly didactic teaching; in others, programs extend to 40 h and include theoretical lessons, case discussions, and high-fidelity simulation [54–56]. Teaching formats are likewise highly variable: In some curricula, frontal teaching predominates, whereas in others, practical components and simulation account for a substantial proportion of the program [54–56].

Continuing education is also characterized by marked heterogeneity. Broadly speaking, two predominant models can be identified, whose effectiveness has never been compared in robust studies. The first is the "one-time training" model: Nurses receive initial training, after which no structured updates are provided [57]. This approach rests on an implicit assumption that competence remains stable over time, an assumption not supported by the available evidence and indeed contradicted by numerous studies in other clinical domains, such as resuscitation, which document substantial skill decay within 6–12 months of training.

The second model, which may be termed "continuous education," provides periodic updates, but with highly variable frequency, duration, and content [58]. In some contexts, brief annual sessions focused on selected updates are offered; in others, more structured quarterly programs of around 8 h are implemented. In most cases, content is determined locally, in the absence of a shared framework, and evaluation of the effectiveness of educational interventions is either absent or sporadic.

This situation contrasts sharply with areas such as basic life support and defibrillation (BLS-D), where international protocols define with precision the recommended retraining interval, course duration, minimum mandatory content based on standardized algorithms, and methods of assessment through structured skill tests [59]. For triage, by contrast, no analogous reference framework currently exists.

7.4.1 The Paradox of Experience: Contradictory Findings

One of the most debated issues in the triage literature concerns the role of clinical experience. Some studies support the notion that greater seniority in the emergency department is associated with higher accuracy, whereas others find no correlation or even report opposite associations [21, 57, 60, 61].

These apparent contradictions can be explained, at least in part, by several mechanisms. First, many studies do not adequately control for confounding factors such as specific triage training, the complexity of the cases assigned, and potential selection bias (e.g., nurses with poorer performance who leave the triage role).

Second, a further element is the lack of structured feedback: In many settings, experience accumulates without any systematic mechanism for reviewing and correcting errors, favoring the consolidation of suboptimal decision patterns. The concept of the "experienced non-expert," well described in the psychology of expertise, highlights that simple repetition is insufficient to build advanced competence in the absence of guided deliberate practice [51]. Finally, methodological variability across studies, with differing definitions of "experience" and heterogeneous performance measures, hampers comparison and contributes to the fragmentation of results.

Overall, the available literature does not allow definitive conclusions to be drawn regarding the role of experience. This uncertainty represents a substantial methodological failure: After decades of triage research, we still do not know with sufficient confidence whether, and in what way, experience influences performance, precisely because education and evaluation have not been adequately standardized.

7.4.2 Gaps in Evaluating the Clinician Rather Than the System

The vast majority of publications address the validity and reliability of the systems themselves, whereas only a small proportion directly examines education or competence, and a similar proportion investigates organizational factors [5, 6].

This bias has important consequences. When a system shows suboptimal performance in terms of under-triage, over-triage, or sensitivity for critical conditions, problems tend to be attributed to the system per se, and new versions or alternative models are proposed [5, 6]. Much less attention is paid to the possibility that a substantial share of the variance may depend on the operator or the context. This generates a vicious circle: Faced with unsatisfactory performance, a new system is introduced, implemented without adequate training and without modifying the organizational setting, performance remains poor, and yet another system change is advocated.

To accurately identify targets for intervention, triage performance must be deconstructed into its main components. A conceptual framework can be proposed in which performance is a function of four factors: the system, the operator, the context, and their interaction. The system includes characteristics such as the number of urgency levels, the presence and quality of discriminators, and the structure of decision algorithms. The operator encompasses education, experience, clinical competence, fatigue, and cognitive biases. The context refers to available resources, crowding, time pressure, and technological support. The interaction reflects the degree of fit between system and operator, practical usability, and integration within the workflow.

To fully appreciate the magnitude of the educational gap in triage, it is useful to compare this field with others in which standardization has been achieved. In basic life support and defibrillation, for example, initial training typically lasts 8 h; retraining is mandatory every 2 years; course content is defined by shared international guidelines; and assessment is based on written tests and practical skills evaluations with clearly specified pass criteria [59, 62, 63]. The result is a substantial global uniformity in basic resuscitation competencies.

In triage, by contrast, initial training ranges from 4 to 40 h, often without a shared core curriculum; retraining is absent or left to the discretion of individual institutions or triage systems; content depends on local systems and trainers' preferences; no international certification exists; and assessment is heterogeneous or, at times, entirely lacking. Despite more than 50 years of modern triage practice, fragmentation remains the defining feature of education and competency standards in this domain.

7.4.3   Consequences of Fragmented Training

The lack of standardization in training makes it extremely difficult to conduct robust comparative research between institutions, systems, or countries. When comparing the performance of two departments that use, for example, ATS and ESI, differences in reliability coefficients or under-triage rates cannot be attributed unequivocally to the system itself, because multiple confounding factors intervene: differing duration and structure of training programs, epidemiological case-mix, availability of diagnostic resources, and organizational culture. Without a minimum common training denominator, such comparisons are methodologically weak.

Fragmentation also hinders the development of international collaborative networks [2]. Nurses trained on different systems often do not share a common conceptual language, which makes the exchange of best practices and the joint design of research projects more difficult. In other areas, such as trauma or sepsis, international courses and campaigns have provided a shared frame of reference that facilitates collaboration and interoperability; in triage, this common foundation is lacking.

Each institution or system is forced to develop its own teaching materials, training programs, and assessment tools, resulting in enormous duplication of effort and cost. The consequence is inefficient use of resources, with programs that frequently replicate very similar content without proportional gains in quality. Supra-national standardization would allow development costs to be shared, improve the quality of materials, and free resources for research and innovation.

In conclusion, the training of triage nurses currently represents one of the major gaps both in triage practice and in triage research. While we possess extensive evidence on system validation, we still know little about how to train staff effectively and maintain their competencies over time. This asymmetry has tangible consequences: persistent inter-operator variability, uncertainty regarding the role of experience, difficulty in conducting robust comparative studies, and, ultimately, risks to patient safety.

International standardization of training, inspired by successful models such as BLS-D, is not utopian but a concrete possibility, provided there is political will, adequate investment, collaboration among scientific societies, institutions and professionals, and a commitment to generating solid evidence on the effectiveness of educational interventions.

Triage is too important to be left to the current degree of variability. Every patient, regardless of where they present and which clinician assesses them, has the right to accurate and safe triage. Standardizing triage nurse education is the indispensable foundation for achieving this objective.

References

1. Fry M, Stainton C. An educational framework for triage nursing based on gatekeeping, time-keeping and decision-making processes. Accid Emerg Nurs. 2005;13(4):214–9. https://doi.org/10.1016/j.aaen.2005.09.004.
2. Zaboli A. Establishing a common ground: the future of triage systems. BMC Emerg Med. 2024;24(1):148. https://doi.org/10.1186/s12873-024-01070-2.
3. Fekonja Z, Kmetec S, Fekonja U, Mlinar Reljić N, Pajnkihar M, Strnad M. Factors contributing to patient safety during triage process in the emergency department: a systematic review. J Clin Nurs. 2023;32(17–18):5461–77. https://doi.org/10.1111/jocn.16622.
4. Christ M, Grossmann F, Winter D, Bingisser R, Platz E. Modern triage in the emergency department. Dtsch Arztebl Int. 2010;107(50):892–8. https://doi.org/10.3238/arztebl.2010.0892.
5. Hinson JS, Martinez DA, Cabral S, et al. Triage performance in emergency medicine: a systematic review. Ann Emerg Med. 2019;74(1):140–52. https://doi.org/10.1016/j.annemergmed.2018.09.022.
6. Zachariasse JM, van der Hagen V, Seiger N, Mackway-Jones K, van Veen M, Moll HA. Performance of triage systems in emergency care: a systematic review and meta-analysis. BMJ Open. 2019;9(5):e026471. https://doi.org/10.1136/bmjopen-2018-026471.
7. Nishi FA, Polak C, Cruz DALMD. Sensitivity and specificity of the Manchester triage system in risk prioritization of patients with acute myocardial infarction who present with chest pain. Eur J Cardiovasc Nurs. 2018;17(7):660–6. https://doi.org/10.1177/1474515118777402.

8. Hoo ZH, Candlish J, Teare D. What is an ROC curve? Emerg Med J. 2017;34(6):357–9. https://doi.org/10.1136/emermed-2017-206735.

9. Streiner DL, Cairney J. What's under the ROC? An introduction to receiver operating characteristics curves. Can J Psychiatr. 2007;52(2):121–8. https://doi.org/10.1177/070674370705200210.

10. Challen K. How good is triage, and what is it good for? Emerg Med J. 2017;34(11):702. https://doi.org/10.1136/emermed-2017-206973.

11. Moll HA. Challenges in the validation of triage systems at emergency departments. J Clin Epidemiol. 2010;63(4):384–8. https://doi.org/10.1016/j.jclinepi.2009.07.009.

12. Kuriyama A, Urushidani S, Nakayama T. Five-level emergency triage systems: variation in assessment of validity. Emerg Med J. 2017;34(11):703–10. https://doi.org/10.1136/emermed-2016-206295.

13. Evans C, Hughes C, Ferguson J. Improving patient safety through the introduction of a formal triage process. Emerg Nurse. 2017;24(9):19–25. https://doi.org/10.7748/en.2017.e1647.

14. Huabbangyang T, Rojsaengroeng R, Tiyawat G, et al. Associated factors of under and over-triage based on the emergency severity index; a retrospective Cross-sectional study. Arch Acad Emerg Med. 2023;11(1):e57. Published 2023 Aug 21. https://doi.org/10.22037/aaem.v11i1.2076.

15. Parenti N, Reggiani ML, Iannone P, Percudani D, Dowding D. A systematic review on the validity and reliability of an emergency department triage scale, the Manchester Triage System. Int J Nurs Stud. 2014;51(7):1062–9. https://doi.org/10.1016/j.ijnurstu.2014.01.013.

16. Hodge A, Hugman A, Varndell W, Howes K. A review of the quality assurance processes for the Australasian triage scale (ATS) and implications for future practice. Australas Emerg Nurs J. 2013;16(1):21–9. https://doi.org/10.1016/j.aenj.2012.12.003.

17. Kemp K, Mertanen R, Lääperi M, Niemi-Murola L, Lehtonen L, Castren M. Nonspecific complaints in the emergency department - a systematic review. Scand J Trauma Resusc Emerg Med. 2020;28(1):6. Published 2020 Jan 28. https://doi.org/10.1186/s13049-020-0699-y.

18. Quinn K, Herman M, Lin D, Supapol W, Worster A. Common diagnoses and outcomes in elderly patients who present to the emergency department with non-specific complaints. CJEM. 2015;17(5):516–22. https://doi.org/10.1017/cem.2015.35.

19. Brutschin V, Kogej M, Schacher S, Berger M, Gräff I. The presentational flow chart "unwell adult" of the Manchester triage system-curse or blessing? PLoS One. 2021;16(6):e0252730. Published 2021 Jun 3. https://doi.org/10.1371/journal.pone.0252730.

20. Nemec M, Koller MT, Nickel CH, et al. Patients presenting to the emergency department with non-specific complaints: the Basel non-specific complaints (BANC) study. Acad Emerg Med. 2010;17(3):284–92. https://doi.org/10.1111/j.1553-2712.2009.00658.x.

21. Ausserhofer D, Zaboli A, Pfeifer N, et al. Errors in nurse-led triage: an observational study. Int J Nurs Stud. 2021;113:103788. https://doi.org/10.1016/j.ijnurstu.2020.103788.

22. Smith J, Filmalter C, Masenge A, Heyns T. The accuracy of nurse-led triage of adult patients in the emergency Centre of urban private hospitals. Afr J Emerg Med. 2022;12(2):112–6. https://doi.org/10.1016/j.afjem.2022.02.007.

23. Suamchaiyaphum K, Jones AR, Markaki A. Triage accuracy of emergency nurses: an evidence-based review. J Emerg Nurs. 2024;50(1):44–54. https://doi.org/10.1016/j.jen.2023.10.001.

24. Zaboli A, Battisti D, Ziller M, Turcato G, Camporesi S. Can patients' characteristics influence triage errors? A Quasi-Experimental study. Int Emerg Nurs. 2025;81:101647. https://doi.org/10.1016/j.ienj.2025.101647.

25. Chen W, Linthicum B, Argon NT, et al. The effects of emergency department crowding on triage and hospital admission decisions. Am J Emerg Med. 2020;38(4):774–9. https://doi.org/10.1016/j.ajem.2019.06.039.

26. Reay G, Smith-MacDonald L, Then KL, Hall M, Rankin JA. Triage emergency nurse decision-making: incidental findings from a focus group study. Int Emerg Nurs. 2020;48:100791. https://doi.org/10.1016/j.ienj.2019.100791.

27. Grossmann FF, Zumbrunn T, Frauchiger A, Delport K, Bingisser R, Nickel CH. At risk of undertriage? Testing the performance and accuracy of the emergency severity index in

older emergency department patients. Ann Emerg Med. 2012;60(3):317–25.e3. https://doi.org/10.1016/j.annemergmed.2011.12.013.

28. Zaboli A, Brigo F, Sibilio S, et al. What is the optimal outcome for evaluating the triage systems? Insights from a prospective observational study. Int Emerg Nurs. 2025;78:101540. https://doi.org/10.1016/j.ienj.2024.101540.

29. Ebrahimi M, Heydari A, Mazlom R, Mirhaghi A. The reliability of the Australasian triage scale: a meta-analysis. World J Emerg Med. 2015;6(2):94–9. https://doi.org/10.5847/wjem.j.1920-8642.2015.02.002.

30. Olofsson P, Gellerstedt M, Carlström ED. Manchester Triage in Sweden – interrater reliability and accuracy. Int Emerg Nurs. 2009;17(3):143–8. https://doi.org/10.1016/j.ienj.2008.11.008.

31. Mistry B, Stewart De Ramirez S, Kelen G, et al. Accuracy and reliability of emergency department triage using the emergency severity index: an international multicenter assessment. Ann Emerg Med. 2018;71(5):581–587.e3. https://doi.org/10.1016/j.annemergmed.2017.09.036.

32. Coronado BE, Pope JH, Griffith JL, Beshansky JR, Selker HP. Clinical features, triage, and outcome of patients presenting to the ED with suspected acute coronary syndromes but without pain: a multicenter study. Am J Emerg Med. 2004;22(7):568–74. https://doi.org/10.1016/j.ajem.2004.09.001.

33. van der Wulp I, Schrijvers AJ, van Stel HF. Predicting admission and mortality with the emergency severity index and the Manchester triage system: a retrospective observational study. Emerg Med J. 2009;26(7):506–9. https://doi.org/10.1136/emj.2008.063768.

34. Lin D, Worster A. Predictors of admission to hospital of patients triaged as nonurgent using the Canadian triage and acuity scale. CJEM. 2013;15(6):353–8. https://doi.org/10.2310/8000.2013.130842.

35. Anesi GL, Admon AJ, Halpern SD, Kerlin MP. Understanding irresponsible use of intensive care unit resources in the USA. Lancet Respir Med. 2019;7(7):605–12. https://doi.org/10.1016/S2213-2600(19)30088-8.

36. Sax DR, Warton EM, Mark DG, Reed ME. Emergency department triage accuracy and delays in care for high-risk conditions. JAMA Netw Open. 2025;8(5):e258498. Published 2025 May 1. https://doi.org/10.1001/jamanetworkopen.2025.8498.

37. Platts-Mills TF, Travers D, Biese K, et al. Accuracy of the emergency severity index triage instrument for identifying elder emergency department patients receiving an immediate life-saving intervention. Acad Emerg Med. 2010;17(3):238–43. https://doi.org/10.1111/j.1553-2712.2010.00670.x.

38. Gräff I, Latzel B, Glien P, Fimmers R, Dolscheid-Pommerich RC. Validity of the Manchester triage system in emergency patients receiving life-saving intervention or acute medical treatment-a prospective observational study in the emergency department. J Eval Clin Pract. 2019;25(3):398–403. https://doi.org/10.1111/jep.13030.

39. Storm-Versloot MN, Vermeulen H, van Lammeren N, Luitse JS, Goslings JC. Influence of the Manchester triage system on waiting time, treatment time, length of stay and patient satisfaction; a before and after study. Emerg Med J. 2014;31(1):13–8. https://doi.org/10.1136/emermed-2012-201099.

40. Cicolo EA, Nishi FA, Peres HHC, Cruz DALMD. Effectiveness of the Manchester triage system on time to treatment in the emergency department: a systematic review. JBI Evid Synth. 2020;18(1):56–73. https://doi.org/10.11124/JBISRIR-2017-003825.

41. Byrne RA, Rossello X, Coughlan JJ, et al. 2023 ESC guidelines for the management of acute coronary syndromes. Eur Heart J Acute Cardiovasc Care. 2024;13(1):55–161. https://doi.org/10.1093/ehjacc/zuad107.

42. Rao SV, O'Donoghue ML, Ruel M, et al. 2025 ACC/AHA/ACEP/NAEMSP/SCAI guideline for the Management of Patients with acute coronary syndromes: a report of the American College of Cardiology/American Heart Association Joint Committee on Clinical Practice Guidelines. Circulation. 2025;151(13):e771–862. https://doi.org/10.1161/CIR.0000000000001309.

43. Yoon P, Steiner I, Reinhardt G. Analysis of factors influencing length of stay in the emergency department. CJEM. 2003;5(3):155–61. https://doi.org/10.1017/s1481803500006539.

44. van der Veen D, Remeijer C, Fogteloo AJ, Heringhaus C, de Groot B. Independent determinants of prolonged emergency department length of stay in a tertiary care centre: a prospective cohort study. Scand J Trauma Resusc Emerg Med. 2018;26(1):81. Published 2018 Sep 20. https://doi.org/10.1186/s13049-018-0547-5.

45. Zaboli A, Pfeifer N, Solazzo P, et al. Blood sampling during nurse triage reduces patient length of stay in the emergency department: a propensity score-weighted, population-based study. Int Emerg Nurs. 2020;49:100826. https://doi.org/10.1016/j.ienj.2019.100826.

46. Chi CH, Huang CM. Comparison of the emergency severity index (ESI) and the Taiwan Triage System in predicting resource utilization. J Formos Med Assoc. 2006;105(8):617–25. https://doi.org/10.1016/S0929-6646(09)60160-1.

47. Lee JY, Oh SH, Peck EH, et al. The validity of the Canadian Triage and Acuity Scale in predicting resource utilization and the need for immediate life-saving interventions in elderly emergency department patients. Scand J trauma Resusc Emerg Med. 2011;19:68. Published 2011 Nov 3. https://doi.org/10.1186/1757-7241-19-68.

48. Mirhaghi A. Resources utilization may not accurately reflect the validity of triage scales. Pediatr Emerg Care. 2025;41(10):e163–4. https://doi.org/10.1097/PEC.0000000000003437.

49. Sember M, Donley C, Eggleston M. Implementation of a provider in triage and its effect on left without being seen rate at a community trauma center. Open Access Emerg Med. 2021;13:137–41. Published 2021 Mar 29. https://doi.org/10.2147/OAEM.S296001.

50. Bambi S, Scarlini D, Becattini G, Alocci P, Ruggeri M. Characteristics of patients who leave the ED triage area without being seen by a doctor: a descriptive study in an urban level II Italian university hospital. J Emerg Nurs. 2011;37(4):334–40. https://doi.org/10.1016/j.jen.2010.05.004.

51. Zaboli A, Sibilio S, Magnarelli G, et al. Daily triage audit can improve nurses' triage stratification: a pre-post study. J Adv Nurs. 2023;79(2):605–15. https://doi.org/10.1111/jan.15521.

52. Zaboli A, Brigo F, Cipriano A, et al. Assessing triage efficiency in Italy: a comparative study using simulated cases among nurses. Intern Emerg Med. 2025;20(4):1167–76. https://doi.org/10.1007/s11739-024-03735-z.

53. Mustafa MA, Al-Khafaji ZAT, Al-Hussien IQK. Challenges and knowledge of nurses regarding triage systems in emergency departments. Malays J Nurs. 2025;17(Suppl 1):100–11.

54. Rankin JA, Then KL, Atack L. Can emergency nurses' triage skills be improved by online learning? Results of an experiment. J Emerg Nurs. 2013;39(1):20–6. https://doi.org/10.1016/j.jen.2011.07.004.

55. Shin HJ, Park S, Lee HJ. Optimizing triage education for emergency room nurses: a scoping review. Nurse Educ Today. 2025;144:106452. https://doi.org/10.1016/j.nedt.2024.106452.

56. McNally S. The triage role in emergency nursing: development of an educational programme. Int J Nurs Pract. 1996;2(3):122–8. https://doi.org/10.1111/j.1440-172x.1996.tb00037.x.

57. Zaboli A, Brigo F, Magnarelli G, et al. Reproducibility of the Manchester Triage System: a multicentre vignette study. Emerg Med J. 2025;42(6):403–10. Published 2025 May 22. https://doi.org/10.1136/emermed-2024-214213.

58. Hinds A, Kay S, Evans K. Refresher training for emergency department triage nurses – a scoping review. Australas Emerg Care. 2025;28(3):204–12. https://doi.org/10.1016/j.auec.2025.03.006.

59. Woollard M, Whitfield R, Newcombe RG, Colquhoun M, Vetter N, Chamberlain D. Optimal refresher training intervals for AED and CPR skills: a randomised controlled trial. Resuscitation. 2006;71(2):237–47. https://doi.org/10.1016/j.resuscitation.2006.04.005.

60. Cetin SB, Eray O, Cebeci F, Coskun M, Gozkaya M. Factors affecting the accuracy of nurse triage in tertiary care emergency departments. Turk. J Emerg Med. 2020;20(4):163–7. Published 2020 Oct 7. https://doi.org/10.4103/2452-2473.297462.

61. Hwang S, Shin S. Factors affecting triage competence among emergency room nurses: a cross-sectional study. J Clin Nurs. 2023;32(13–14):3589–98. https://doi.org/10.1111/jocn.16441.
62. Hsieh MJ, Chiang WC, Jan CF, Lin HY, Yang CW, Ma MH. The effect of different retraining intervals on the skill performance of cardiopulmonary resuscitation in laypeople-a three-armed randomized control study. Resuscitation. 2018;128:151–7. https://doi.org/10.1016/j.resuscitation.2018.05.010.
63. Hamilton R. Nurses' knowledge and skill retention following cardiopulmonary resuscitation training: a review of the literature. J Adv Nurs. 2005;51(3):288–97. https://doi.org/10.1111/j.1365-2648.2005.03491.x.

What Can Be Improved in the Short-Term Future and for the Long-Term Future of Triage Systems

8

Over the last 20 years, triage systems have established themselves as the universal language of urgency [1]. The shared objective across international experiences has been to translate the initial clinical impression into a codified operational priority capable of ensuring consistency, timeliness, and safety in decision-making [2, 3]. This methodological coherence has produced robust results, with good levels of discriminative accuracy for clinically relevant outcomes such as short-term critical events, need for hospital admission, or urgent interventions [2, 3].

However, when viewed through the lens of predictive statistics, triage systems reveal a structural limitation that is both technical and conceptual. In most of the available evidence, the discriminatory power of triage systems is expressed by AUROC values around 0.70–0.75: results that indicate a good ability to distinguish patients who will experience adverse outcomes from those who will not, but that remain distant from theoretical excellence [3, 4]. In practical terms, this means that triage is reliable but not infallible: There is a "predictive gap," a missing 0.3 that separates real-world performance from theoretical perfection [3, 4].

This gap should not be interpreted as an intrinsic weakness of the systems, but rather as the reflection of a clinical complexity that is not fully captured by the variables on which current triage models are based. The architecture of these systems, although accurate, focuses predominantly on the acute dimension of clinical presentation: symptoms, vital signs, level of consciousness, and pattern of onset. Yet what the system does not observe, or cannot observe in the limited time available at arrival, is far from irrelevant: biological and functional frailty, cumulative comorbidity, physiological reserve, social vulnerability, and the capacity of the organism to withstand acute stress [5–7]. These elements, which profoundly influence prognosis, largely remain outside the triage process or are considered only intuitively, without a structured translation into operational decisions [5–7].

In other words, triage measures the urgency of the event with precision but does not always capture the patient's resilience in the face of that event. It evaluates current severity, but not the probability of deterioration. The literature has shown that,

A. Zaboli, G. Turcato, *Triage Systems: Essential Knowledge for Emergency Nurses and Physicians*, https://doi.org/10.1007/978-3-032-20825-5_8

for the same initial presentation, patients with frailty or multiple comorbidities have significantly worse outcomes: higher risk of ICU admission, early mortality, and hospital readmission. Yet these vulnerability factors are still not systematically embedded in triage methodologies [5–9].

The goal, therefore, is not to replace existing models, but to increase their cognitive resolution. Like an image sharpened by adding additional focal planes, triage can evolve by integrating, alongside the assessment of urgency, a broader reading of the patient's overall vulnerability. In this way, prognostic depth, currently confined to the clinician's tacit expertise, can be brought back into the initial decision-making moment. The objective is not to slow triage or overload it with new scales, but to introduce a small number of variables with high predictive yield.

From a Monodimensional Moment to a Multidimensional View of Triage

The "discrimination gap" that separates triage systems from predictive excellence is not merely a technical limitation; it is an opportunity for transformation. It represents the possibility of evolving from a monodimensional view of triage, centered exclusively on immediate priority, to a multidimensional perspective capable of integrating, alongside urgency, the patient's biological and functional complexity and other physiopathological dimensions of the underlying condition [10].

In its original conception, triage was designed as a rapid and uniform sorting device, created primarily to satisfy an organizational need rather than a prognostic one: determining who should be seen first. The increasing complexity of patients, population aging, multimorbidity, and growing pressure on health services now demand a conceptual leap in triage itself, which must become the starting point of prediction, not only of classification.

Within the brief interval between the patient's arrival and the first decision, the highest time-value information of the entire care pathway is concentrated. In this narrow window, clinical perception, expert intuition, and objective tools can work together to generate a robust initial prediction. Multidimensionality does not mean adding more data but interpreting existing data more effectively, cross-referencing them with indicators of vulnerability, functional reserve, and evolutionary risk.

Overcoming a monodimensional view of triage entails abandoning the linear logic of "symptom equal priority" and adopting a perspective that conceptualizes risk as a multidimensional function arising from the interaction between the acute event and the patient's individual characteristics [10]. Thinking of triage in multimodal terms means broadening the decision horizon: not only "who is worse now" but also "who is most likely to deteriorate soon." This should not make the process heavier, but rather more refined: triage as the junction between classification and prediction, between urgency and vulnerability.

The evolution toward multidimensional triage can follow two main operational directions, both already explored in the modern international literature: internal integration and sequential integration.

In the internal integration model, extended assessment elements, such as composite physiological scores, frailty indices, rapid instrumental parameters, or focused clinical tools, are incorporated directly into the triage process [10–12]. This approach reduces informational discontinuity, enabling the professional to construct a more complete picture of the patient from the very first contact. Its main advantage is cognitive continuity: The triage nurse retains control of the entire decision flow, transforming clinical perception into a structured and documented risk estimate.

However, this model requires advanced expertise, rigorous protocol governance, and well-defined activation criteria in order to prevent the cognitive expansion from degenerating into subjective variability or operational slowdown. The core challenge is to balance depth and speed, integrating without overburdening, enriching without dispersing focus.

In the sequential integration model, by contrast, multidimensional assessment is placed in an immediately subsequent module, performed in continuity by the same team or in dedicated spaces [13]. The urgency level assigned by the triage system becomes only one of the dimensions explored in this "triage moment." Alongside urgency, it must be possible to examine other domains that contribute to predicting the patient's true risk in terms that are no longer merely classificatory but genuinely prognostic [13, 14].

This configuration preserves the rapidity and lightness of the initial act while allowing more in-depth early stratification in complex cases. It is a flexible model, suitable for high-volume settings with diversified resources, where the second assessment phase can be activated selectively according to predefined risk criteria: advanced age, relevant comorbidities, and signs of subclinical instability. In this way, cognitive overload for the triage nurse is avoided and flow remains fluid, while achieving more accurate prediction. At the same time, however, the model inevitably loses some of the speed and narrow focus on "urgency only" and becomes broader and more generalist, requiring substantially greater human and structural resources.

Both models converge toward a hybrid perspective, in which the choice between internal or sequential integration is not alternative but adaptive. In a truly evolved system, triage could incorporate a small set of essential risk indicators directly into the assignment flow, while other elements are collected in an early stratification module activated according to case complexity. The future of triage will therefore be hybrid and dynamic, able to combine the speed of classification with the depth of prediction.

Conceptualizing triage as a "cognitive space" means no longer viewing it as a mere algorithm, but as a decision context with maximal information density. In that brief time interval, the professional can blend clinical perception, probabilistic reasoning, and decision-support tools to formulate a robust initial forecast. Multidimensionality is not an accumulation of data, but a shift in perspective: learning to read simultaneously urgency, severity, complexity, reserve, and context.

In this view, the clinician's experience, guided by structured systems, is not replaced by tools but amplified. Standardized instruments do not crowd out intuition; they render it verifiable and reproducible by anchoring it to objective criteria.

Adopting a multidimensional perspective also demands cultural and organizational evolution. For decades, the quality of triage has been measured in terms of speed and inter-observer agreement; tomorrow, the most meaningful metric may be overall predictive capacity. The key question is no longer how quickly a code is assigned, but how accurately that rapid code predicts clinical risk and influences patient outcomes.

This implies a redefinition of the competencies required of triage nurses, who must be able to recognize early indicators of deterioration, interpret physiopathological patterns, and use rapid but information-rich tools, such as ECG or venous blood gas analysis, not merely as technical acts to shorten timelines, but as components of an early, comprehensive, and above all autonomous prognostic assessment.

At the same time, organizations must create flexible operational spaces, shared protocols, and information systems capable of integrating data collected at triage into the clinical workflow in real time. The deepest transformation, however, remains cognitive. It means shifting from a logic of priority to a logic of prediction: no longer asking only "whom should I see first?" but also "who is most likely to deteriorate if I do not intervene immediately?"

Multidimensional triage does not negate the original function of triage; it completes it. It acknowledges that apparent severity is only one component of real risk and that each patient carries a potential trajectory that must be anticipated rather than merely observed. From this perspective, bridging the 0.3 gap does not mean pursuing an abstract mathematical ideal of perfection, but restoring triage to its deepest clinical essence: transforming reception into prediction, classification into understanding, and speed into clinical intelligence.

8.1   Multimodal Assessment of the Patient at Triage

The multidimensional perspective on triage is grounded in the idea that urgency is never the product of a single axis, but the result of a complex interaction between the acute event and the patient's profile. Each individual brings a unique combination of factors that modulate the response to physiological stress, the speed of deterioration, and therefore the probability of adverse outcomes.

However, the current structure of triage systems, oriented toward simplification and rapidity, captures only part of this complexity. What remains outside, baseline biology, functional frailty, physiological reserves, adaptive capacity, constitutes exactly that quota of information that could transform a purely classificatory assessment into a more accurate predictive estimate. Integrating these elements at the triage stage does not mean overloading nursing practice with new procedures; rather, it means bringing back into the clinical scene elements already present in the mind of the experienced professional and translating them into a shared, structured language.

Within this framework, additional major predictive domains, closely interconnected with urgency, can be identified: comorbidity, illness intensity, ands frailty. Each offers a complementary perspective and helps to bridge the gap between the snapshot of the acute event and an understanding of the patient's clinical trajectory.

8.1.1   Comorbidity

Comorbidity represents the chronic dimension of risk. It is not simply a list of diagnoses, but a system of pathological interactions that profoundly alters the organism's response to acute stress [15, 16]. The impact of an acute illness cannot be evaluated without taking into account the biological "terrain" on which it occurs.

A patient with ischemic heart disease, chronic obstructive pulmonary disease, and chronic kidney disease does not respond to the same clinical insult in the same way as a previously healthy individual: The compensatory margin is smaller, organ reserve is more fragile, and the probability of decompensation is higher. Numerous studies have shown that cumulative comorbidity is one of the strongest determinants of in-hospital mortality and intensive care admission, independent of apparent severity at presentation [15–18].

Yet this information enters the triage process only indirectly, through the presenting symptom, and not as an intrinsic characteristic of the individual patient. The clinical history, often scattered across information systems or only partially reported by the patient, remains at the margins of assessment. This leads to a loss of critical information: Two patients with the same triage code may have very different outcome risks purely because of their different comorbidity burden.

Integrating comorbidity into triage does not necessarily mean constructing new, complex scales, but rather recognizing the existence of high-risk patterns and training clinicians to identify them rapidly.

Comorbidity is thus less a single variable and more a lens through which the acute illness can be interpreted within its biological context.

8.1.2   Illness Intensity: The Pathophysiological Depth of the Event

The second, often underestimated, dimension is illness intensity. This is not the perceived severity of the symptom, a severe pain does not necessarily equate to high risk, but the pathophysiological depth of the acute disturbance. Intensity reflects the extent to which the acute process has already compromised vital functions or how much reserve remains before compensation fails [19].

In traditional triage, severity is often estimated on the basis of macroscopic signs: vital parameters, level of consciousness, skin color, and sweating. However, there are conditions in which impairment is subclinical: early sepsis, a still-compensated internal hemorrhage, incipient respiratory failure [19]. In these cases, assessing illness intensity makes it possible to anticipate the trajectory of deterioration before it becomes overt.

From this perspective, the triage nurse must refine the ability to detect weak signals: subtle changes in respiratory rate, a barely borderline oxygen saturation in a patient with limited reserve, and the appearance of minimal behavioral changes in an older person. Technology can amplify this sensitivity through the use of synthetic physiological scores such as National Early Warning Scores or Modified Early

Warning Score, which can be calculated in a few seconds and allow the physiological intensity of the event to be quantified and translated into a shared language [19–22]. Illness intensity therefore represents the dynamic dimension of risk. Although some triage systems already take it into account for specific symptomatic presentations, its systematic incorporation into the initial assessment could strengthen the prognostic value of triage.

8.1.3 Frailty

Frailty is perhaps the subtlest, and at the same time the most decisive, dimension of risk. It does not coincide with comorbidity or chronological age; rather, it describes a condition of global biological vulnerability, a reduced capacity to maintain homeostasis in the face of even minimal stress. A frail person is not simply an elderly patient, but an organism with diminished functional reserve, limited biological resources, and chronic metabolic and immune alterations that amplify the impact of any acute insult [23].

Frailty explains why two apparently similar patients, with the same symptom and the same vital signs, may experience very different clinical trajectories. It is a cross-cutting risk modifier that acts on every dimension of acute illness: time to decompensation, therapeutic response, and capacity for recovery [23, 24]. Yet in traditional triage, frailty remains invisible because it is not immediately measurable. In recent years, several rapid screening tools have been developed, such as the Clinical Frailty Scale or PRISMA-7, which allow intrinsically more vulnerable patients to be identified within a few seconds [11, 25]. Recent studies have shown that adding a simple frailty assessment at triage improves predictive accuracy for adverse outcomes [26].

Even when it is not formally measured, frailty can be recognized through macroscopic behavioral or functional indicators. Incorporating frailty into the initial assessment therefore represents a decisive step towards a more personalized and individualized emergency medicine.

These dimensions, urgency, comorbidity, intensity, and frailty, do not operate independently; they are interwoven in a complex mosaic that can define the patient's predictive and risk profile at the moment of triage. Considering them separately serves only analytical purposes, because in clinical reality they amplify one another.

Multimodal assessment does not aim to create new categories, but to offer a cognitive framework for interpreting complexity. Each domain can be explored with simple tools, sometimes purely observational, but the key is integration. Within this logic, the triage nurse becomes the first observer of the overall risk, the professional who constructs a synthetic yet meaningful representation of the patient.

Operationally, translating these concepts into practice may take different forms: enhancing existing triage systems by integrating these dimensional spheres into decision-making processes, or creating, within the triage encounter, dedicated spaces, protocols, and tools capable of linking the urgency level assigned by the triage system to these additional dimensions.

8.2   Rapid Clinical Tools to Improve Triage

In addition to deepening the different dimensions of the patient who presents to triage with an acute symptom, with the aim of improving overall risk prediction within a multidimensional framework, contemporary emergency medicine now has access to high-yield clinical tools. These are characterized by high discriminatory and diagnostic power, are easily accessible, and can be rapidly deployed in everyday practice. One need only consider the capacity of a 12-lead electrocardiogram (ECG) to direct early suspicion toward an acute coronary syndrome in the presence of chest pain, or the use of symptom-specific clinical scores that can guide, from the very first minutes, either suspicion or exclusion of a particular disease.

Over the last decade, a substantial body of scientific work has demonstrated that critical-care and emergency nurses possess the competencies required to use tools traditionally considered the exclusive domain of physicians, such as ECG interpretation, or blood gas analysis. These skills, now widely established in nursing practice, have been progressively recognized also within triage operations themselves, to the point that, in some local contexts, such tools are already formally integrated into triage protocols as codified operational components [27, 28].

Several recent studies have further shown that nurses, through the use of targeted clinical tools, can safely up- or downgrade the urgency level assigned by the triage system, thereby improving the precision with which high-risk patients are discriminated [27, 28]. Both the direct integration of such tools into triage systems and their use immediately after code assignment have proved feasible and effective, improving overall performance and increasing triage sensitivity in the early recognition of critically ill patients.

In parallel with multimodal assessment, the use of clinical instruments and tools can likewise be conceived from a dual perspective: integrated into the triage systems themselves, in order to enhance predictive performance in specific symptomatic conditions, or applied immediately after code assignment, enabling the nurse to complete the "triage moment" with a more in-depth evaluation of the patient's overall risk profile.

8.2.1   Electrocardiogram: From Technical Test to Early Predictive Device

In the triage setting, the 12-lead electrocardiogram is not merely a traditional diagnostic test, but a potential modulator of the system's discriminatory capacity. International guidelines for the management of chest pain explicitly recommend performing an ECG within 10 min of arrival for patients presenting with chest pain, recognizing that the timeliness of this examination constitutes a quality indicator for the entire time-sensitive care pathway [29, 30].

Observational studies and quality-improvement projects have shown that organizational strategies centered on early ECG acquisition on nurse initiative at triage significantly reduce door-to-ECG times and, consequently, door-to-balloon times in patients with coronary disease, with favorable associations in terms of outcomes and the proportion of patients treated within recommended time windows [31]. In this sense, an ECG performed at the time of triage is not an ancillary act, but a key step that injects very high-density prognostic information into the initial decision-making window.

The structured incorporation of ECG into triage can address two converging needs. On the one hand, it makes it possible to reduce under-triage of cardiac patients by detecting early atypical STEMI, NSTEMI with subtle symptoms, major arrhythmias, or electrical signs of instability that may not be accompanied by a dramatically obvious clinical picture. Studies on dedicated cardiac triage models and on nurse-initiated immediate ECG protocols show more appropriate assignment of priority codes and earlier identification of high-risk patients, with a measurable impact on timeliness of care [32, 33].

On the other hand, the ECG is one of the core components of major chest-pain stratification tools (such as HEART score), which integrate clinical history, risk factors, ECG findings, and biomarkers to estimate the risk of major adverse cardiac events (MACE) and to support rapid decisions regarding referral to high-intensity pathways or, conversely, safe discharge in low-risk patients [34, 35]. Including ECG within the "triage moment," or within a structured assessment module that follows immediately and is tightly integrated with it, therefore strengthens triage as the first level of cardiac risk prediction, transforming it from a purely symptom-based device into a platform capable of linking clinical presentation, electrocardiographic evidence, and time-critical pathways [36].

From a professional standpoint, the literature supports the role of the triage nurse as a competent actor in initiating, promoting, and managing early ECG acquisition, showing that focused educational interventions and nurse-initiated protocols significantly improve system performance without increasing false positives or overloading patient flow. Multiple studies underscore that nurses are fully capable of reading the ECG and interpreting it within the context of an acute presentation, thereby enhancing their predictive ability for risk in patients with cardiac problems [36–38].

In this perspective, the ECG becomes the paradigmatic example of how a simple, widely available tool, if intentionally placed at the right point in the process, namely, triage, can increase the system's sensitivity for high-risk patients and contribute concretely to closing part of the discriminatory gap that currently characterizes triage systems.

8.2.2   Blood Gas Analysis at Triage: Making Physiological Reserve Visible and Anticipating Risk

In the context of early risk stratification, blood gas analysis, arterial or venous, particularly in a point-of-care format, represents a tool with very high predictive value, capable of transforming an apparently stable clinical picture into an objective assessment of physiological reserve [39–41]. Unlike simple vital signs, which describe only the surface of the problem, blood gas analysis directly measures acid–base balance, ventilation, oxygenation, and tissue metabolism, allowing early identification of patients who are already "paying the price" of significant metabolic or respiratory stress [39–41].

Numerous studies have highlighted the prognostic value of early lactate measurement: Elevated lactate levels at triage are associated with an independent increase in short-term mortality and in the need for intensive treatments [42, 43]. Capillary lactate measurement performed in triage has also proved technically feasible and strongly correlated with adverse outcomes, supporting its use as a high-priority indicator to distinguish, among clinically similar patients, those who require accelerated pathways [42].

Beyond lactate, blood gas analysis has a targeted role in acute respiratory syndromes and in exacerbations of COPD or heart failure, where it enables rapid differentiation between patients who can be safely managed in lower-intensity settings and those with acidosis, hypercapnia, or gas-exchange abnormalities that herald an imminent risk of respiratory failure. In sepsis, protocols that include early lactate measurement show a strong correlation with 48-h and 28-day mortality, supporting the use of blood gas analysis as an early warning and monitoring tool in patients with suspected subclinical instability [44, 45].

Evidence also shows that nurses who are adequately trained are able to interpret blood gas results correctly, correlating parameters such as pH, $PaCO_2$, PaO_2, and lactate with the clinical picture and anticipating the risk of respiratory or metabolic deterioration [46]. Autonomous interpretation of blood gas analysis can thus function as an early signal of instability, adding a measurable physiological dimension to clinical perception.

The effectiveness of blood gas analysis at triage, however, depends on its appropriate use. Indiscriminate testing increases costs and workload without real benefit, whereas selective use, based on nurse-initiated protocols for dyspnea, suspected shock, sepsis, or altered mental status, allows immediate incorporation of results into priority assignment and care pathways. From this perspective, blood gas analysis is not a routine test but a high-specificity predictive tool, capable of illuminating the grey zones of clinical risk at an early stage and contributing concretely to reducing the discriminatory gap of current triage systems.

8.2.3   The Use of Clinical Scores in Triage

In recent years, emergency medicine has progressively recognized that risk prediction cannot rely solely on qualitative judgements or rigid thresholds for vital signs. In a context where decisions must be taken within minutes, often with incomplete information, clinical scores represent one of the most powerful methodological evolutions: They transform clinical perception into a structured probabilistic estimate.

In triage, their function is not to replace the judgement of the clinician operating within a given system, but to provide objective tools capable of reducing variability between professionals and settings, offering a quantitative measure of risk that can complement subjective assessment. Scores are synthetic instruments that combine clinical, physiological, or laboratory variables into mathematical models able to express a probability of adverse events. Their diffusion in emergency medicine stems from the need to anchor decisions to actual risk and not merely to momentary clinical impression.

At the time of triage, when uncertainty is greatest and time is shortest, the application of validated scores makes it possible to anticipate the patient's clinical trajectory and to direct diagnostic and therapeutic pathways with greater precision [47, 48]. Recent literature emphasizes that integrating scores into the triage phase improves the discriminatory capacity of traditional systems. In several meta-analyses, the addition of indices such as NEWS2, MEWS, or qSOFA to standard triage parameters has produced a significant increase in AUROC for prediction of mortality and rapid deterioration [49–51].

These tools offer the advantage of encoding a symptomatic pattern in a simple and rapid way, transforming it into a reproducible estimate that can be communicated among clinicians. The use of scores at triage should therefore be understood not as an extra "checklist" but as a numerical language of complexity that becomes a shared alphabet. When applied in the appropriate context, each score refines risk perception, corrects cognitive bias, and improves concordance between nursing assessment and medical decision-making. In addition, scores allow monitoring of clinical dynamics over time, enabling structured reassessments based on changes in physiological parameters or worsening symptoms.

Several triage systems already include vital signs in their architecture as key elements for assigning urgency level; some, such as the Emergency Severity Index (ESI) and the Australasian Triage Scale (ATS), base their initial discrimination precisely on the combination of respiratory rate, mental status, and signs of physiological compromise. However, simple measurement of these parameters, if not structured, risks remaining a static snapshot rather than a dynamic measure of risk.

Integrating a physiological score alongside the traditional scale allows the clinician to pair bedside judgement with a numerical index of objective risk that does not replace the decision but becomes its measurable and shareable extension. In this way, the numerical component reduces inter-observer variability, increases consistency of decisions among professionals, and strengthens clinical communication within the multidisciplinary team. The result is a more predictive triage, capable of blending the sensitivity of clinical experience with the statistical robustness of physiological assessment tools.

It is important to underline that not all scores are equivalent. Some, such as NEWS, are based on universal physiological parameters and provide a transversal assessment of severity [49–51]. Others, such as Emergency Department Assessment of Chest Pain (EDACS), or scores for syncope and sepsis, are symptom-specific and follow a logic of targeted prediction centered on a particular clinical domain [47, 52, 53]. Both families of tools, physiological and disease-specific, can be integrated into the "triage moment," but with different purposes: the former to define global risk, the latter to guide diagnostic probability and the need for immediate investigations.

The incorporation of these instruments into triage therefore represents a crucial step in the transition from reactive to predictive medicine. It means moving from urgency classification based on the present to dynamic stratification that considers the patient's near clinical future. In this sense, scores are not an operational constraint but an amplifier of clinical judgement, helping clinicians to see beyond the appearance of stability and detect the weak signals of imminent instability.

8.3   Artificial Intelligence

Artificial intelligence (AI) represents one of the most promising and, at the same time, most controversial frontiers in the evolution of triage systems. The possibility of using advanced algorithms to support clinical risk stratification, reduce inter-operator variability, and optimize patient flow in Emergency Departments has generated, in recent years, unprecedented scientific and commercial interest. This enthusiasm has, however, been accompanied by substantial methodological confusion, inappropriate applications of available technologies, and, in some cases, futuristic visions that fail to recognize the fundamental nature of the triage process and the irreplaceable competencies of health professionals.

The present section aims to provide a critical, evidence-based perspective on the role of artificial intelligence in triage, distinguishing, on the one hand, between appropriate and promising applications and, on the other, methodologically problematic or conceptually flawed approaches.

To understand the potential role of AI in triage, it is essential to distinguish between different technological architectures and their appropriate fields of application.

8.3.1   Machine Learning and Deep Learning: Appropriate Foundations

Supervised machine learning currently represents the most established and methodologically appropriate approach for clinical applications in triage [54]. It is based on training algorithms on large datasets of clinical cases with known outcomes, on the selection and transformation of predictive clinical variables, on rigorous performance validation using independent test cohorts, and on the possibility of interpreting, at least in part, the factors that drive predictions [55]. Among the most frequently used algorithms are logistic regression, which enables the prediction of binary outcomes through linear models; random forests, which combine numerous decision trees to handle complex non-linear relationships; gradient boosting machines, optimized for predictive accuracy; and support vector machines, which aim to achieve optimal separation between classes [55, 56].

Deep learning, a subcategory of machine learning based on deep artificial neural networks, offers particularly relevant capabilities for the analysis of complex and unstructured data [55, 57]. Its distinctive features include the ability to automatically learn the most relevant features without manual feature engineering, the effective handling of high-dimensional data, and the construction of hierarchical representations of patterns with progressively higher levels of abstraction [55, 57].

8.3.2 Generative AI: Limitations and Unsuitability for Clinical Triage

A specific class of artificial intelligence systems, generative AI, and in particular large language models (LLMs), such as ChatGPT, Gemini, Copilot, and others, has demonstrated impressive performance in linguistic and creative tasks [58, 59]. However, these systems have structural limitations that render them unsuitable for critical clinical applications such as triage.

From an architectural standpoint, LLMs are intrinsically probabilistic and non-deterministic: Given the same input, they may generate different outputs in successive runs [58, 59]. This variability is incompatible with the requirements for reproducibility and standardization that are essential for a clinical triage system. Studies reported wide variability in the clinical recommendations produced by the same model for identical clinical cases, suggesting substantial unreliability when standardized decisions are required [60, 61].

Moreover, LLMs do not operate through genuine, structured clinical reasoning, but through statistical recognition of textual patterns. They do not possess an understanding of pathophysiology, do not apply diagnostic algorithms in a systematic way, and do not follow clinical protocols consistently. Added to this is the phenomenon of so-called "hallucinations": the generation of linguistically plausible but factually incorrect information [62, 63]. Such errors are unacceptable in the triage context. A further limitation is the lack of reliable probabilistic calibration, which prevents associating recommendations with clinically meaningful estimates of uncertainty.

8.3.3 Confusion in the Recent Literature

In the past few years, there has been a rapid proliferation of studies exploring the use of LLMs for triage, but much of this work is affected by substantial methodological limitations [64]. Critical reviews of this emerging field indicate that most evaluations rely on simplified simulated cases or exam-style vignettes that do not reflect the complexity, noise, and incompleteness of real triage encounters [64, 65]. Only a minority of studies use real patient data or compare LLM performance directly with established, validated triage systems [61, 66–68]. In addition, outcomes are frequently surrogate measures, such as agreement with an expert rater or classification accuracy on synthetic scenarios, rather than patient-centered safety endpoints like adverse events, time-critical treatment, or resource use [61, 66–68].

The result is an evidence base crowded with findings described as "promising" but built on fragile designs. This risks creating conceptual confusion, diverting attention away from more robust approaches to decision support and encouraging premature implementation of LLM-based tools in clinical triage, with potential implications for patient safety.

8.3.4   The Indispensable Value of Bedside Clinical Judgement

Triage is a complex clinical process that integrates multiple sources of information, many of which are not easily digitized. Direct observation during the first seconds of contact provides an immediate impression of the patient's overall condition: skin color and perfusion, degree of sweating, posture and movement patterns, facial expression, respiratory effort, and psychomotor state. These cues often guide the initial estimation of risk before any formal measurement is taken [69, 70].

Targeted physical examination further refines this assessment. In trauma, palpation, inspection, and brief neurological checks can reveal instability or focal deficits that are not yet reflected in vital signs [71, 72]. In abdominal pain, guarding, rebound tenderness, and subtle signs of peritonism are highly informative [72].

Non-verbal communication and the relational context also play a central role. Incongruence between what the patient says and how they appear, for example, minimizing symptoms despite evident distress, is a frequent trigger for re-evaluating risk [73]. Information from relatives or witnesses, recent functional decline, and details of the mechanism of injury further shape the clinical picture. Environmental and social indicators, such as personal care, mode of arrival or signs of social vulnerability, contribute to the overall assessment and are difficult to capture in structured digital fields.

These components, which are integral to how experienced triage nurses think and decide, remain largely inaccessible to current AI systems.

8.3.5   The Problem with Self-Triage and Fully Automated Triage

Proposals for fully automated triage or patient self-triage, sometimes assisted by AI tools, raise major conceptual and empirical concerns [74, 75]. By definition, patients in true emergency conditions are often in pain, distressed, hypoxic or cognitively impaired, and therefore poorly positioned to judge their own urgency.

Studies on digital symptom checkers and self-triage tools consistently show a combination of under-triage of high-risk patients and over-triage of minor conditions, with only moderate agreement with clinician-assigned urgency levels [74, 76]. The resulting noise limits their usefulness as a stand-alone gatekeeper for access to emergency departments [76].

Beyond accuracy, there is a risk that such systems could distort the mission of emergency services. Patients with serious conditions might be discouraged from attending because an automated tool has labelled them as "non-urgent," while individuals with minor complaints but greater digital literacy could obtain disproportionate priority. This dynamic would weaken the safety-net function of professional triage, whose role includes detecting unrecognized vulnerability, picking up on subtle deterioration in patients with low health literacy, and providing orientation and reassurance.

From a medico-legal standpoint, the allocation of responsibility for errors made by autonomous self-triage systems remains unclear, creating additional risk for healthcare organizations.

8.3.6   The Appropriate Model: AI as Decision Support

A more realistic and safe paradigm for AI in triage is the clinical decision support system (CDSS). In this model, algorithms provide recommendations that clinicians can accept, modify, or reject, with their rationale documented.

A well-designed CDSS for triage is fed with structured inputs: demographic information, standardized reason for visit, complete vital signs, key symptoms captured through validated checklists, mechanism of injury, medication history, and allergies [77, 78]. These data are processed by machine-learning models trained on large datasets and integrated with existing validated triage scales [77–79]. Contextual factors such as crowding and resource availability can also be incorporated to support situational awareness.

The output should be interpretable. Instead of a black-box decision, the system should suggest a priority level with an accompanying confidence estimate, highlight the variables that most influenced the recommendation, flag possible time-critical conditions, and indicate when additional assessments are advisable. Crucially, the clinician must retain the ability to override the recommendation, with reasons recorded. Systematic analysis of these overrides, linked to outcomes, can be used both to evaluate clinical judgement and to iteratively refine the algorithm.

When implemented in this way, decision-support tools in emergency care have been associated with improved recognition of time-sensitive conditions, reductions in under-triage and more consistent use of escalation pathways, without unacceptable increases in over-triage or loss of professional autonomy [78, 79].

8.3.7   Specific Benefits of AI-Assisted Triage

If embedded as decision support, AI can contribute in several ways. Algorithms that systematically re-evaluate the full set of available data may help counter anchoring, premature closure, and other common biases, especially by prompting reconsideration when new or discordant information appears [80, 81].

Moreover, during crowding and long shifts, AI tools can maintain vigilance by issuing alerts for high-risk patterns, reminding staff of scheduled re-assessments, and ensuring that key fields are not left undocumented [81, 82].

Lastly, comparing clinician decisions with model recommendations and subsequent outcomes can offer powerful feedback on calibration of risk perception, particularly for rare or complex presentations [83].

In all these roles, AI amplifies rather than replaces the clinical reasoning of the triage nurse.

8.3.8 Requirements for Safe and Effective Implementation

Safe integration of AI into triage demands stringent technical, clinical, and organizational conditions.

From a technical perspective, models should be trained on large, representative datasets and validated on independent cohorts from different institutions [54]. Performance must be at least comparable to that of existing validated triage systems, and fairness analyses across demographic groups are essential to detect and correct potential inequities.

From a clinical perspective, prospective evaluations in multiple emergency departments are needed, with outcomes that reflect patient safety, such as short-term mortality, unplanned ICU admission, and serious adverse events, rather than purely statistical metrics. Usability and acceptance by clinicians should be assessed alongside accuracy, as poor integration into workflow can negate theoretical benefits.

From an implementation-governance perspective, AI-based triage support should be treated as a medical device where regulations require, with clear accountability, continuous post-implementation monitoring, defined procedures for reporting incidents linked to the system, and periodic re-evaluation on real-world data. Multidisciplinary governance structures should oversee model updates, override policies and audit processes, and ensure that staff feedback is systematically collected and acted upon.

8.3.9 Training and Change Management

Introducing AI into triage also requires substantial investment in education and change management. Clinicians need a basic literacy in AI: understanding how models are developed, what their outputs mean, how confidence scores and risk thresholds work, and what typical failure modes look like.

These competencies should be incorporated into undergraduate curricula and reinforced through continuing education, simulation exercises that include decision-support tools, and periodic assessments of appropriate use. Organizationally, involving frontline clinicians in design and local adaptation, using user-centered interface design, piloting systems with structured feedback loops, and appointing local clinical champions are all crucial to sustainable adoption.

8.3.10 Concluding Perspective

The scientific, clinical, and regulatory communities should resist the temptation to deploy immature technologies driven by hype or commercial pressure. The history of medicine is rich in examples of promising tools that, when implemented prematurely, failed to improve outcomes, or even caused harm, delaying the adoption of genuinely useful innovations.

It is likely that the future of triage will see increasing integration with AI systems. That future will be beneficial only if it is built on robust evidence, respect for clinical expertise, commitment to equity and, above all, an unwavering focus on patient safety. The goal for the coming decade is not to replace triage nurses, but to design AI systems that make them more effective; not to bypass clinical judgement, but to strengthen it; not to widen disparities, but to help close them. Ultimately, AI-assisted triage should serve the core mission of emergency care: ensuring that every patient receives the right level of care, at the right time, regardless of who they are or where they come from.

References

1. Zaboli A. Establishing a common ground: the future of triage systems. BMC Emerg Med. 2024;24(1):148. Published 2024 Aug 15. https://doi.org/10.1186/s12873-024-01070-2.
2. Kuriyama A, Urushidani S, Nakayama T. Five-level emergency triage systems: variation in assessment of validity. Emerg Med J. 2017;34(11):703–10. https://doi.org/10.1136/emermed-2016-206295.
3. Hinson JS, Martinez DA, Cabral S, et al. Triage performance in emergency medicine: a systematic review. Ann Emerg Med. 2019;74(1):140–52. https://doi.org/10.1016/j.annemergmed.2018.09.022.
4. Zachariasse JM, van der Hagen V, Seiger N, Mackway-Jones K, van Veen M, Moll HA. Performance of triage systems in emergency care: a systematic review and meta-analysis. BMJ Open. 2019;9(5):e026471. Published 2019 May 28. https://doi.org/10.1136/bmjopen-2018-026471.
5. Boreskie PE, Boreskie KF. Frailty-aware care in the emergency department. Emerg Med Clin North Am. 2025;43(2):199–210. https://doi.org/10.1016/j.emc.2024.08.004.
6. van Dam CS, Labuschagne HA, van Keulen K, et al. Polypharmacy, comorbidity and frailty: a complex interplay in older patients at the emergency department. Eur Geriatr Med. 2022;13(4):849–57. https://doi.org/10.1007/s41999-022-00664-y.
7. Rivers E, Nguyen B, Havstad S, et al. Early goal-directed therapy in the treatment of severe sepsis and septic shock. N Engl J Med. 2001;345(19):1368–77. https://doi.org/10.1056/NEJMoa010307.
8. Sert ET, Kokulu K, Mutlu H, Yortanlı BC. Effects of clinical frailty scale score on adverse outcomes and length of emergency department stay before intensive Care unit admission. J Emerg Med. 2024;66(1):e10–9. https://doi.org/10.1016/j.jemermed.2023.08.020.
9. Liu H, Song B, Jin J, et al. Length of stay, hospital costs and mortality associated with comorbidity according to the Charlson comorbidity index in immobile patients after ischemic stroke in China: a National Study. Int J Health Policy Manag. 2022;11(9):1780–7. 10.34172/ijhpm.2021.79
10. Zaboli A, Brigo F, Sibilio S, et al. An alternative perspective on triage systems: the Progressive Real-world Optimization of Triage System (PROGRESS) study. Emerg Care J. 2025;21(2):e13269. https://doi.org/10.4081/ecj.2025.13269.
11. Chung HS, Choi Y, Lim JY, et al. Validation of the Korean version of the clinical frailty scale-adjusted Korean triage and acuity scale for older patients in the emergency department. Medicina (Kaunas). 2024;60(6):955. Published 2024 Jun 8. https://doi.org/10.3390/medicina60060955.

12. Lin PC, Wu MY, Chien DS, et al. Use of reverse shock index multiplied by simplified motor score in a five-level triage system: identifying trauma in adult patients at a high risk of mortality. Medicina (Kaunas). 2024;60(4):647. Published 2024 Apr 18. https://doi.org/10.3390/medicina60040647.

13. Zaboli A, Sibilio S, Magnarelli G, Pfeifer N, Brigo F, Turcato G. Development and validation of a nomogram for assessing comorbidity and frailty in triage: a multicentre observational study. Intern Emerg Med. 2024;19(8):2249–58. https://doi.org/10.1007/s11739-024-03593-9.

14. Zaboli A, Sibilio S, Brigiari G, et al. External validation of the TFC (triage frailty and comorbidity) tool: a prospective observational study. Intern Emerg Med. 2025;20(4):1195–202. https://doi.org/10.1007/s11739-024-03757-7.

15. Olsson T, Terent A, Lind L. Charlson comorbidity index can add prognostic information to rapid emergency medicine score as a predictor of long-term mortality. Eur J Emerg Med. 2005;12(5):220–4. https://doi.org/10.1097/00063110-200510000-00004.

16. Bahrmann A, Benner L, Christ M, et al. The Charlson comorbidity and Barthel index predict length of hospital stay, mortality, cardiovascular mortality and rehospitalization in unselected older patients admitted to the emergency department. Aging Clin Exp Res. 2019;31(9):1233–42. https://doi.org/10.1007/s40520-018-1067-x.

17. Donatelli NS, Gregorowicz J, Somes J. Extended ED stay of the older adult results in poor patient outcome. J Emerg Nurs. 2013;39(3):268–72. https://doi.org/10.1016/j.jen.2013.02.005.

18. Murray SB, Bates DW, Ngo L, Ufberg JW, Shapiro NI. Charlson Index is associated with one-year mortality in emergency department patients with suspected infection. Acad Emerg Med. 2006;13(5):530–6. https://doi.org/10.1197/j.aem.2005.11.084.

19. Howell MD, Donnino MW, Talmor D, Clardy P, Ngo L, Shapiro NI. Performance of severity of illness scoring systems in emergency department patients with infection. Acad Emerg Med. 2007;14(8):709–14. https://doi.org/10.1197/j.aem.2007.02.036.

20. Zaboli A, Brigo F, Sibilio S, et al. Evaluating the National Early Warning Score (NEWS) in triage: a machine learning perspective. Int Emerg Nurs. 2025;80:101602. https://doi.org/10.1016/j.ienj.2025.101602.

21. Keep JW, Messmer AS, Sladden R, et al. National early warning score at Emergency Department triage may allow earlier identification of patients with severe sepsis and septic shock: a retrospective observational study. Emerg Med J. 2016;33(1):37–41. https://doi.org/10.1136/emermed-2014-204465.

22. Schinkel M, Bergsma L, Veldhuis LI, Ridderikhof ML, Holleman F. Comparing complaint-based triage scales and early warning scores for emergency department triage. Emerg Med J. 2022;39(9):691–6. https://doi.org/10.1136/emermed-2021-211544.

23. Gordon EH, Peel NM, Hubbard RE, Reid N. Frailty in younger adults in hospital. QJM. 2023;116(10):845–9. https://doi.org/10.1093/qjmed/hcad173.

24. Wolf LA, Lo AX, Serina P, et al. Frailty assessment tools in the emergency department: a geriatric emergency department guidelines 2.0 scoping review. J Am Coll Emerg Physicians Open. 2023;5(1):e13084. Published 2023 Dec 29. https://doi.org/10.1002/emp2.13084.

25. O'Caoimh R, McGauran J, O'Donovan MR, et al. Frailty screening in the emergency department: comparing the variable indicative of placement risk, clinical frailty scale and PRISMA-7. Int J Environ Res Public Health. 2022;20(1):290. Published 2022 Dec 24. https://doi.org/10.3390/ijerph20010290.

26. Zaboli A, Brigo F, Brigiari G, et al. Comparative analysis of frailty scales in emergency department: highlighting the strengths of the triage frailty and comorbidity tool. J Emerg Nurs. 2025;51(1):135–44. https://doi.org/10.1016/j.jen.2024.09.012.

27. Alwosibei A, Alqurashi H, Alghazwi M. Role of venous blood gas (VBG) analysis in patient triage in the adult emergency department. JMLPH. 2023;3(3):277–81. https://doi.org/10.52609/jmlph.v3i3.83.

28. Zaboli A, Sibilio S, Brigo F, et al. The triage nurse's ability in electrocardiogram interpretation in real clinical practice. J Clin Nurs. 2023;32(15–16):4904–14. https://doi.org/10.1111/jocn.16624.

29. Gulati M, Levy PD, Mukherjee D, et al. AHA/ACC/ASE/CHEST/SAEM/SCCT/SCMR guideline for the evaluation and diagnosis of CHEST pain: a report of the American College of Cardiology/American Heart Association Joint Committee on Clinical Practice Guidelines. Circulation. 2021;144(22):e368–454. https://doi.org/10.1161/CIR.0000000000001029.

30. Gulati M, Levy PD, Mukherjee D, et al. 2021 AHA/ACC/ASE/CHEST/SAEM/SCCT/SCMR guideline for the evaluation and diagnosis of CHEST pain: executive summary: a report of the American College of Cardiology/American Heart Association Joint Committee on Clinical Practice Guidelines. Circulation. 2021;144(22):e368–454. https://doi.org/10.1161/CIR.0000000000001030.

31. Chhabra S, Eagles D, Kwok ESH, Perry JJ. Interventions to reduce emergency department door-to- electrocardiogram times: a systematic review. CJEM. 2019;21(5):607–17. https://doi.org/10.1017/cem.2019.342.

32. Nishi FA, Polak C, Cruz DALMD. Sensitivity and specificity of the Manchester Triage System in risk prioritization of patients with acute myocardial infarction who present with chest pain. Eur J Cardiovasc Nurs. 2018;17(7):660–6. https://doi.org/10.1177/1474515118777402.

33. Atzema CL, Austin PC, Tu JV, Schull MJ. ED triage of patients with acute myocardial infarction: predictors of low acuity triage. Am J Emerg Med. 2010;28(6):694–702. https://doi.org/10.1016/j.ajem.2009.03.010.

34. Backus BE, Six AJ, Kelder JC, et al. A prospective validation of the HEART score for chest pain patients at the emergency department. Int J Cardiol. 2013;168(3):2153–8. https://doi.org/10.1016/j.ijcard.2013.01.255.

35. Laureano-Phillips J, Robinson RD, Aryal S, et al. HEART score risk stratification of low-risk chest pain patients in the emergency department: a systematic review and meta-analysis. Ann Emerg Med. 2019;74(2):187–203. https://doi.org/10.1016/j.annemergmed.2018.12.010.

36. Zaboli A, Ausserhofer D, Sibilio S, et al. Electrocardiogram interpretation during nurse triage improves the performance of the triage system in patients with cardiovascular symptoms – a prospective observational study. Int Emerg Nurs. 2023;68:101273. https://doi.org/10.1016/j.ienj.2023.101273.

37. Coll-Badell M, Jiménez-Herrera MF, Llaurado-Serra M. Emergency nurse competence in electrocardiographic interpretation in Spain: a cross-sectional study. J Emerg Nurs. 2017;43(6):560–70. https://doi.org/10.1016/j.jen.2017.06.001.

38. Ho JK, Yau CH, Wong CY, Tsui JS. Capability of emergency nurses for electrocardiogram interpretation. Int Emerg Nurs. 2021;54:100953. https://doi.org/10.1016/j.ienj.2020.100953.

39. Tienpratarn W, Yuksen C, Chukaew L, Jenpanitpong C, Triganjananun C, Seesuklom S. Point-of-Care Testing (POCT) for blood gas and electrolyte analysis in out-of-hospital cardiac arrests' management; a cross-sectional study. Arch Acad Emerg Med. 2025;13(1):e32. Published 2025 Jan 25. https://doi.org/10.22037/aaemj.v13i1.2590.

40. Walther LH, Zegers F, Nybo M, et al. Accuracy of a point-of-care blood lactate measurement device in a prehospital setting. J Clin Monit Comput. 2022;36(6):1679–87. https://doi.org/10.1007/s10877-022-00812-6.

41. Pradhan J, Harding AM, Taylor SE, Lam Q. Implications of differences between point-of-care blood gas analyser and laboratory analyser potassium results on hyperkalaemia diagnosis & treatment. Intern Med J. 2023;53(11):2035–41. https://doi.org/10.1111/imj.16020.

42. Fukumoto Y, Inoue Y, Takeuchi Y, et al. Utility of blood lactate level in triage. Acute Med Surg. 2015;3(2):101–6. Published 2015 Aug 17. https://doi.org/10.1002/ams2.130.

43. Datta D, Walker C, Gray AJ, Graham C. Arterial lactate levels in an emergency department are associated with mortality: a prospective observational cohort study. Emerg Med J. 2015;32(9):673–7. https://doi.org/10.1136/emermed-2013-203541.

44. Bhat SR, Swenson KE, Francis MW, Wira CR. Lactate clearance predicts survival among patients in the emergency department with severe sepsis. West J Emerg Med. 2015;16(7):1118–26. https://doi.org/10.5811/westjem.2015.10.27577.

45. Shapiro NI, Howell MD, Talmor D, et al. Serum lactate as a predictor of mortality in emergency department patients with infection. Ann Emerg Med. 2005;45(5):524–8. https://doi.org/10.1016/j.annemergmed.2004.12.006.

46. Zaboli A, Biasi C, Magnarelli G, et al. Arterial blood gas analysis and clinical decision-making in emergency and intensive care unit nurses: a performance evaluation. Healthcare (Basel). 2025;13(3):261. Published 2025 Jan 28. https://doi.org/10.3390/healthcare13030261.

47. Zaboli A, Ausserhofer D, Sibilio S, et al. Effect of the emergency department assessment of chest pain score on the triage performance in patients with chest pain. Am J Cardiol. 2021;161:12–8. https://doi.org/10.1016/j.amjcard.2021.08.058.

48. Ng ALY, Yeo CHX, Ong ST, et al. Improving triage accuracy through a modified nurse-administered emergency department assessment of chest pain score on patients with chest pain at triage (EDACT): a prospective observational study. Int Emerg Nurs. 2022;61:101130. https://doi.org/10.1016/j.ienj.2021.101130.

49. Saberian P, Tavakoli N, Hasani-Sharamin P, Modabber M, Jamshididana M, Baratloo A. Accuracy of the pre-hospital triage tools (qSOFA, NEWS, and PRESEP) in predicting probable COVID-19 patients' outcomes transferred by emergency medical services. Caspian. J Intern Med. 2020;11(Suppl 1):536–43. https://doi.org/10.22088/cjim.11.0.536.

50. Kemp K, Alakare J, Harjola VP, et al. National Early Warning Score 2 (NEWS2) and 3-level triage scale as risk predictors in frail older adults in the emergency department. BMC Emerg Med. 2020;20(1):83. Published 2020 Oct 28. https://doi.org/10.1186/s12873-020-00379-y.

51. Prasad PA, Fang MC, Martinez SP, Liu KD, Kangelaris KN. Identifying the sickest during triage: using point-of-care severity scores to predict prognosis in emergency department patients with suspected sepsis. J Hosp Med. 2021;16(8):453–61. https://doi.org/10.12788/jhm.3642.

52. Nieves Ortega R, Rosin C, Bingisser R, Nickel CH. Clinical scores and formal triage for screening of sepsis and adverse outcomes on arrival in an emergency department all-comer cohort. J Emerg Med. 2019;57(4):453–460.e2. https://doi.org/10.1016/j.jemermed.2019.06.036.

53. Del Rosso A, Ungar A, Maggi R, et al. Clinical predictors of cardiac syncope at initial evaluation in patients referred urgently to a general hospital: the EGSYS score. Heart. 2008;94(12):1620–6. https://doi.org/10.1136/hrt.2008.143123.

54. Levin S, Toerper M, Hamrock E, et al. Machine-learning-based electronic triage more accurately differentiates patients with respect to clinical outcomes compared with the emergency severity index. Ann Emerg Med. 2018;71(5):565–574.e2. https://doi.org/10.1016/j.annemergmed.2017.08.005.

55. Ramlakhan S, Saatchi R, Sabir L, et al. Understanding and interpreting artificial intelligence, machine learning and deep learning in emergency medicine. Emerg Med J. 2022;39(5):380–5. https://doi.org/10.1136/emermed-2021-212068.

56. Couronné R, Probst P, Boulesteix AL. Random forest versus logistic regression: a large-scale benchmark experiment. BMC Bioinformatics. 2018;19(1):270. Published 2018 Jul 17. https://doi.org/10.1186/s12859-018-2264-5.

57. Sidey-Gibbons JAM, Sidey-Gibbons CJ. Machine learning in medicine: a practical introduction. BMC Med Res Methodol. 2019;19(1):64. Published 2019 Mar 19. https://doi.org/10.1186/s12874-019-0681-4.

58. Deng J, Zubair A, Park YJ, Affan E, Zuo QK. The use of large language models in medicine: proceeding with caution. Curr Med Res Opin. 2024;40(2):151–3. https://doi.org/10.1080/03007995.2023.2295411.

59. Choi J. Large language models in medicine. Healthc Inform Res. 2025;31(2):111–3. https://doi.org/10.4258/hir.2025.31.2.111.

60. Bruce J. White coat oversight of black-box algorithms: ethical challenges in the application of Artificial Intelligence in Healthcare. J Med Law Public Health. 2025;5(4):782–90. https://doi.org/10.52609/jmlph.v5i3.216.

61. Zaboli A, Brigo F, Sibilio S, Mian M, Turcato G. Human intelligence versus Chat-GPT: who performs better in correctly classifying patients in triage? Am J Emerg Med. 2024;79:44–7. https://doi.org/10.1016/j.ajem.2024.02.008.

62. Beutel G, Geerits E, Kielstein JT. Artificial hallucination: GPT on LSD? Crit Care. 2023;27(1):148. Published 2023 Apr 18. https://doi.org/10.1186/s13054-023-04425-6.

63. Chelli M, Descamps J, Lavoué V, et al. Hallucination rates and reference accuracy of ChatGPT and bard for systematic reviews: comparative analysis. J Med Internet Res. 2024;26:e53164. Published 2024 May 22. https://doi.org/10.2196/53164.

64. Kaboudi N, Firouzbakht S, Shahir Eftekhar M, et al. Diagnostic accuracy of ChatGPT for Patients' Triage; a systematic review and meta-analysis. Arch Acad Emerg Med. 2024;12(1):e60. Published 2024 Jul 30. https://doi.org/10.22037/aaem.v12i1.2384.

65. Shool S, Adimi S, Saboori Amleshi R, Bitaraf E, Golpira R, Tara M. A systematic review of large language model (LLM) evaluations in clinical medicine. BMC Med Inform Decis Mak. 2025;25(1):117. Published 2025 Mar 7. https://doi.org/10.1186/s12911-025-02954-4.

66. Colakca C, Ergın M, Ozensoy HS, Sener A, Guru S, Ozhasenekler A. Emergency department triaging using ChatGPT based on emergency severity index principles: a cross-sectional study. Sci Rep. 2024;14(1):22106. Published 2024 Sep 27. https://doi.org/10.1038/s41598-024-73229-7.

67. Zaboli A, Brigo F, Brigiari G, et al. Chat-GPT in triage: still far from surpassing human expertise – an observational study. Am J Emerg Med. 2025;92:165–71. https://doi.org/10.1016/j.ajem.2025.03.028.

68. Kim JH, Kim SK, Choi J, Lee Y. Reliability of ChatGPT for performing triage task in the emergency department using the Korean Triage and Acuity Scale. Digit Health. 2024;10:20552076241227132. Published 2024 Jan 17. https://doi.org/10.1177/20552076241227132.

69. Suzuki R, Takada T, Miyashita J, Fukuhara S. Utility of triage nurses' quick-look assessments of adults in the emergency Department for Predicting Hospital Admission. J Emerg Nurs. 2025;51(6):1140–9. https://doi.org/10.1016/j.jen.2025.06.002.

70. Betz M, Stempien J, Wilde A, Bryce R. A comparison of a formal triage scoring system and a quick-look triage approach. Eur J Emerg Med. 2016;23(3):185–9. https://doi.org/10.1097/MEJ.0000000000000239.

71. Jayashree M, Singhi SC. Initial assessment and triage in ER. Indian J Pediatr. 2011;78(9):1100–8. https://doi.org/10.1007/s12098-011-0411-3.

72. Zaboli A, Ausserhofer D, Pfeifer N, et al. Acute abdominal pain in triage: a retrospective observational study of the Manchester triage system's validity. J Clin Nurs. 2021;30(7–8):942–51. https://doi.org/10.1111/jocn.15635.

73. Roscoe LA, Eisenberg EM, Forde C. The role of patients' stories in emergency medicine triage. Health Commun. 2016;31(9):1155–64. https://doi.org/10.1080/10410236.2015.1046020.

74. Lammila-Escalera E, Greenfield G, Aldakhil R, et al. Safety and efficacy of digital check-in and triage kiosks in emergency departments: systematic review. J Med Internet Res. 2025;27:e69528. Published 2025 May 21. https://doi.org/10.2196/69528.

75. Brown HL. evaluation of artificial intelligence for patient self-triage: comparison of general-purpose AI platforms with the NHS 111 online symptom checker in the United Kingdom. Cureus. 2025;17(11):e97834. Published 2025 Nov 26. https://doi.org/10.7759/cureus.97834.

76. Trivedi SV, Batta R, Henao-Romero N, Mondal P, Wilson T, Stempien J. A comparison of self-triage tools to nurse driven triage in the emergency department. PLoS One. 2024;19(8):e0297321. Published 2024 Aug 28. https://doi.org/10.1371/journal.pone.0297321.

77. Tyler S, Olis M, Aust N, et al. Use of artificial intelligence in triage in hospital emergency departments: a scoping review. Cureus. 2024;16(5):e59906. Published 2024 May 8. https://doi.org/10.7759/cureus.59906.

78. Taylor RA, Chmura C, Hinson J, Steinhart B, Sangal R, Venkatesh AK, Xu H, Cohen I, Faustino IV, Levin S. Impact of artificial intelligence–based triage decision support on emergency department care. NEJM AI. 2025;2(3) https://doi.org/10.1056/AIoa2400296.

79. Mejia JMR, Rawat DB. Exploring the advancements of AI enabled clinical decision support systems for patient triage in healthcare. In: 2024 IEEE international conference on E-health networking, application & services (HealthCom); Nara, Japan, vol. 1-4; 2024. https://doi.org/10.1109/HealthCom60970.2024.10880833.

80. Cross JL, Choma MA, Onofrey JA. Bias in medical AI: implications for clinical decision-making. PLOS Digit Health 2024;3(11):e0000651. Published 2024 Nov 7. https://doi.org/10.1371/journal.pdig.0000651.
81. Hinson JS, Levin SR, Steinhart BD, et al. Enhancing emergency department triage equity with artificial intelligence: outcomes from a multisite implementation. Ann Emerg Med. 2025;85(3):288–90. https://doi.org/10.1016/j.annemergmed.2024.10.014.
82. Piliuk K, Tomforde S. Artificial intelligence in emergency medicine. A systematic literature review. Int J Med Inform. 2023;180:105274. https://doi.org/10.1016/j.ijmedinf.2023.105274.
83. Li Y, Jiang S, Dai S, et al. Use of machine learning for risk stratification of chest pain patients in the emergency department. BMC Med Inform Decis Mak. 2025;25(1):393. Published 2025 Oct 24. https://doi.org/10.1186/s12911-025-03226-x.